"Read Dr. Weinberg's book and prepare to experience something wonderful; wisdom written in a very understandable, enlightening, and life-enhancing style. Dr. Barry is a rising star, and I have a feeling this is just the first of many works of wisdom we'll be experiencing from him."

Bob Burg, *Author*
Endless Referrals and Winning Without Intimidation

"In reading Dr. Weinberg's excellent testimony to the power of the human spirit when guided by Love and Caring, I was taken by the very practical and *do-able* tasks outlined in the book. Not only is this a superior summation of what the holistic healing movement stands for, but it gives an easy-to-apply "How to get your body and soul" assignment formula, so that the reader can turn theory into pro-action. I highly recommend this book to anyone who wants to expand their personal health horizons (and have fun doing it!)"

Ron Mercer, *Ph.D., LMHC, NCC*
Co-Director, Center for Effective Living
Psychotherapist / Men's Issues Specialist.

"Follow Dr. Barry's path step-by-step as he leads you through the power of your mind to choose transformation in your life. For one so young to have such depth of feeling for his humanity is a blessing for all of us who have worked with him and experienced his compassion and healing touch. He has illuminated my mind and heart; consequently changes I never thought possible have occurred in my life. His book is a gift to all who read it."

Eleanor R. Caimano, *Business Woman*

"Our family's experience with Dr. Barry is a complete delight. We consider him one of the great healers on the planet and his book is a gift to mankind. We bless him and his wife Anja."

Rabbi and Rebbetzin Yehuda and Margot Greenberg

"This book is a reflection of Dr. Weinberg's extraordinary gift for clarity and sensitivity. I felt 'taken care of' and confident of the research and integrity that went into creating this reference book. I know that I can count on it now and in the future as different needs arise in my life. Thank you for making a difference in the lives of people."

Debbie Schwartz, *Leadership Coach*

A Clear Path to Healing

A Clear Path to Healing

Reclaiming the
Inner Healing Power
of body and mind
to reach your
optimum health potential

Dr. Barry S. Weinberg

Dream Reality Productions, Inc.
Fort Lauderdale, Florida

Cover Design by Dream Reality Productions, Inc.
Cover Photo taken in Utah by Anja Weinberg
Portrait Photo by Jess Hooper

Book design and layout by
Karen Petherick, Markham, ON, Canada

Dr. Barry Weinberg is available as a keynote speaker for seminars and workshops
to any organization. In addition, he encourages those who have studied his book
to form study groups based on A Clear Path to Healing.

Please visit our website at www.placeforhealing.com

ISBN 0-9679360-0-4
Library of Congress Card Number: 00-191442
Manufactured in the United States

Published by Dream Reality Productions, Inc.
Fort Lauderdale, Florida

THIS BOOK IS DEDICATED TO

all those brave souls who
think their own thoughts,
speak their own truth,
and walk their own path,
in spite of the fear they feel.

TABLE OF CONTENTS

PART II OFF THE BEATEN PATH

PART III A CLEAR PATH TO HEALING

ACKNOWLEDGEMENTS

First and foremost, I thank God for my life and the inspiration to write this book. The information contained in this book came through me, but from this source of all things.

I thank my wife Anja for always standing by my side and giving me her love and companionship that keeps me going on my own *clear path to healing*.

I thank my parents and my family who have always allowed me and encouraged me to be the best me I can be.

I thank all my patients and all those I have served at A Place for Healing for teaching me the awesome healing power of the human body and for giving me the opportunity to participate in their healing, growth, and evolution.

I thank Dr. Donald Epstein for being my mentor and coach on my healing journey and teaching me to be the best doctor and healing facilitator I can be.

I thank Bob Proctor for teaching me that my world is a result of my thoughts and empowering me to create a life I had only once dreamed of.

I thank Karen Petherick, for helping to refine my message to its essence. She is the human expression of responsibility and integrity.

I thank my twelfth grade English teacher, Mrs. Sutton, for putting me on the writing path by answering my question, "How long does this report have to be?" with the answer, "Write until you're done." I am still not done.

I would also like to thank all the men and women who have been my teachers through their writings, lectures, and guidance which has given me the knowledge and wisdom to write this book:

Dr. Wayne Dyer, Dr. Deepak Chopra, Neale Donald Walsch, Mayla Makana, Wallace Wattles, Anthony Robbins, Frijof Capra, Ken Wilber, Dan Millman, Daniel Quinn, Og Mandino, Kahlil Gibran, James Ray, James Allen, Napolean Hill, Ralph Waldo Emerson, Dr. Michael Talbot, Jerry and Esther Hicks, Dr. Dennis Perman, Dr. Alan Rousso, Mantak Chia, Paramahansa Yogananda, *The Tao Te Ching, The Bhagavad Gita, The Upanishads, The Holy Bible* and every man, woman, child and animal that I have encountered on this path called Life.

FOREWORD

I believe it was Hubbard who said when you read a good book through the second time, you don't see something in it that you didn't see before, you see something in yourself that wasn't there before. I can guarantee you, this is a book you will go back to a number of times, and on each visit, you will see something new and exciting in yourself. *A Clear Path To Healing* has been designed to draw the very best out of you. Dr. Weinberg is to be congratulated because he has certainly done his homework. It will soon become obvious to you that there has been an enormous amount of research and experience in the preparation of this book. It is virtually an encyclopedia of excellent information on how to live a well-balanced, abundantly healthy life.

After studying human potential and the human personality for close to 40 years, I am totally convinced that the essence of your being is perfect. Brandeis stated that there was a spark of idealism within every human being that could be fanned into flame and would bring extraordinary results. Brandeis was right and the fan required to achieve the results he referred to is understanding. I have found that understanding is the polar opposite to doubt and worry. It is not something that can be inherited or purchased, the only route to develop the understanding you will require to live the "good life" that Dr. Weinberg makes reference to in the introduction is to STUDY and you're certainly on the right track with this book.

I have read thousands of books and studied worldwide for most of my adult life. For over a quarter of a century, Fortune 500 corporations have hired me to teach much of what is in this book to their employees. This information is transformational. Believe me when I tell you it is truly refreshing to have found a book that deals with the primary cause of disease and other aspects of our lives that are unwanted and unnecessary. Most self-help books, books on health and healing focus primarily on treating symptoms. There will never be any permanent change in results in a person's life until they deal with the root cause of the situation they are attempting to change. We have been told to know the truth and the truth would set us free ... there is only one thing to be set free from and that is ignorance. The only way to eliminate ignorance is through knowledge, and the beautiful truth is that you are holding in your hands the knowledge you require to eliminate mountains of ignorance from your life.

Doubt is a mental state that will destroy the mind and body. Dr. Weinberg states very clearly that it is the greatest obstacle on a clear path to healing. He said that as long as doubt is present, nothing is possible. Many years ago, Dr. Mayo from the famous Mayo Clinic said that he had never known anyone to die from overwork, but many who had died from doubt. In the section on doubt, Dr. Weinberg states that what we think creates a vibration that attracts to us whatever is imagined by the thought.

The late Dr. Werhner Von Braun, who is considered by many to be the father of the space program, stated that the natural laws of the universe were so precise that we don't have any difficulty building a spaceship that will carry a man to the moon and we can time the landing with the precision of a fraction of a second. One of those laws is the Law of Vibration that Dr. Weinberg refers to. There are few books that make reference to these laws and yet, the health of your mind and body is going to be determined by your ability to live in harmony with them. You are a spiritual being living in a physical body ... you have been endowed with intellectual factors that enable you to gain an understanding of these laws. Again, it is truly refreshing to see these laws referenced throughout *A Clear Path To Healing*. Long before you finish reading this book, you will be acutely aware that there can be no clear path to healing unless and until you do understand these laws. I have often referred to living in harmony with these laws as getting into the Divine current of life.

Let me caution you, this is not a book that you should be in a hurry to finish reading, rather it is a text that you should enjoy studying. The good life for most of us demands that we alter our paradigm, by internalizing the valuable information on each of these pages you will find your perception of life being altered and your paradigms changed. I am honored that Dr. Weinberg has asked me to share my thoughts with you in the foreword of this book. Permit me to suggest, before you read any further, that you invest in a couple of other copies of this wonderful book and give them to your closest friends. It will be one of the most thoughtful things you can do and it will stimulate meaningful conversation whenever you are with them in the future. Rest assured, all of my friends will have a copy in their library.

Bob Proctor
Fortune 500 Consultant
Best-Selling Author of You Were Born Rich

A CLEAR PATH
TO HEALING

A CLEAR PATH TO HEALING ...

#	Causes of the Health-Care Crisis	Cultural Illusions	Healing Principles	Response Abilities	Powers of the Mind
1	Lack of Responsibility	The Victim	Cause and Effect	Perception	Imagination and Creativity
2	Encouraged Apathy	Possession	Energy and Vibration	Adaptation	Intention and Desire
3	Unwavering Traditionalism	Permanence	Perpetual Change	Recovery	Discrimination and Judgment
4	Nurtured Fear	Helplessness	Inclusive Evolution	Evolution	Belief and Faith
5	Objective Dogma	Scarcity and Failure	Universal Intelligence	Expression	Visualization and Affirmation
6	Separation and Segregation	Separation	Unified Abundance	Harmonious Interaction	Acceptance and Allowance
7	Disempowering Beliefs	The Cure	Subjective Creation	Contentment	Gratitude

... AN OUTLINE

#	Emotions of Dis-ease	Processes of the Heart	Healing Respons-abilities	Individual Benefits	Global Benefits
1	Doubt	Awareness	Positive Mind	Clarity and Peace of Mind	Less Mental Illness and Addiction
2	Apathy	Acknowledgment	Spinal Hygiene	Increased Adaptability to Stress	Stress-Free Society
3	Anxiety	Acceptance	Clean food and Water	Increased Energy and Vitality	Environmental Purity
4	Helplessness	Appreciation	Full, Deep Breathing	Greater Strength and Confidence	Less Physical Disease
5	Sadness	Affirmation	Proper Exercise	Increased Knowledge and Wisdom	Scientific and Technological Advancement
6	Anger	At-One-Ment	A Loving, Giving Heart	Healthy Loving Relationships	Peaceful World Free of Crime and War
7	Fear	Awe	Adequate Rest	Increased Creativity and Prosperity	Increased Prosperity for All

INTRODUCTION

You don't have to be great to get started,
but you do have to get started to be great.
~ Les Brown

*W*hat do you *really* want?

How can I best serve you? What can I do to make this a memorable, life-changing experience? What words will illuminate and enlighten your mind so that when you have finished your journey, your world will be a brighter and happier place? How can I embrace you so that you feel more complete as a result of my touch?

To answer these questions, a deeper issue must be addressed:
What do you want? What do you *really* want?

To have your pain go away? Do you want relief or healing from your ailment, disease or condition? Perhaps, you seek help to handle stress or feel better emotionally? Would you like more energy, increased performance and efficiency in certain tasks or activities?

You may answer yes to one or more of these questions, but is that what you *really* want? Do you really want the pain, disease or problem cured, or is it deeper than that? What is it about your pain – your condition or ailment – that makes you want it to go away? What do you lack or what have you lost that makes you seek assistance to find or regain it?

On the surface you may want these things, but I have found in speaking with thousands of people that what you really want may be something much deeper and much more profound. What most of us really want is *a more joyful, peaceful, love-filled and freer experience of life, and a fuller expression of who we are and the unique gifts we each have to offer the world.*

When you awake each morning, you want to feel secure and safe knowing that the day will be filled with joy, peace and freedom. Each morning, you step out of bed with anticipation that the day holds infinite possibilities for learning, growing and experiencing life to its fullest. Leaving your house, you step outside intent to contribute to the world – to make a difference. And as you return to bed each night, you want to know that today the world is a better place because you were there.

That's what everyone wants ... *really* wants. People want to know that their time spent on this planet makes a difference to others and the world is a better place because they exist upon it.

This is what your pain, ailment or disease takes from you. It is this for which you seek healing. And it is this that I wish to help you experience with this book.

How can I best serve you? By making you aware of the extraordinary power within you.

What is the best thing I can do to make this a memorable, life-changing experience? By helping you discover the wonderful gifts you have to give.

What words can I say to illuminate and enlighten your mind so that when you are finished with this book, your world is a brighter and happier place? You are a powerful being, capable of anything you set your mind to.

How can I embrace you so that you feel more complete as a result of my touch? By showing you a path that is easy and effortless, yet if followed, can give you everything you desire.

It has been said that if you give a person a fish, you feed them for a day, but if you show them how to fish, you feed them for a lifetime. It is my intention to teach you how to fish. Sometimes this can be a little messy, and sometimes down right dirty, however, if you are to be truly free and empowered, and experience complete health, wellness and the joy of life, you need to reach into the belly of the whale and pull out the hook ... yourself.

THE HEALTH-CARE CRISIS

In our country, it is evident that we are in a Health-Care Crisis. The condition of our nation's health and our health-care system has become so critical that it threatens our lives. We are spending more and more money each year on the care of health, yet the American public is getting sicker and sicker.

According to Nancy Dickey, MD, President of the American Medical Association, "Despite huge advances in medical technology and not-withstanding efforts to take advantage of these breakthroughs without raising costs, no one is really happy with the current system. Patients, physicians, the people who pay for health-care all are frustrated. We haven't gotten it right. Our system is out of balance ... It's a mess."[1]

According to the World Health Organization, in 1999, health-care costs have escalated to over $1.2 trillion in the United States, with projections of over $2.2 trillion by the year 2008.[2] With all this spending on health-care, why is it that the incidence of degenerative disease continues to grow? Since 1994, over 35% of the American public suffer from chronic disease, such as cancer, diabetes, arthritis and heart disease, accounting for over 70% of all deaths and 60% of all health-care expenditures in the United States.[3] The United States currently has the finest health-care facilities, the best-trained doctors and the latest cutting-edge, modern technology available in the world, yet the American public is ranked 24th on the World Health Index.[4] The contradiction is readily apparent.

Although this crisis may appear to be of a financial and professional nature, if you look deeper, you will see it is one more personal and esoteric. I believe there are two fundamental causes of this health-care crisis:

- An antiquated mechanistic and materialistic world-view based on an outdated and long disproved science and philosophy.
- A lack of empowerment and responsibility (response ability) on behalf of the individuals of our society.

In this book, it is my intention to present a new, more accurate world-view. One supportive of health and healing – a world-view based upon the enormous personal power of each individual. It is also my intention to provide the knowledge, resources and practical strategy for any individual to accept responsibility for their own life, empowering them to create greater health, happiness and fulfillment in their lives.

A CLEAR PATH TO HEALING

A Clear Path to Healing originally began in the early 1990s with one-hour workshops held in my clinic, local bookstores, and health food stores around town. During these workshops, I taught people how to adopt healthy lifestyle habits in a way that was easy and effortless.

The information I share with you on the following pages remains as I taught it. However, it allows a deeper look into the following:

- the seven causes of the health-care crisis
- the seven healing illusions
- the seven universal principles of healing
- the seven attributes of health
- the seven powers of the mind, and
- the seven processes of the heart
- the seven healing action steps.

Before we begin there is something we must first understand.

WHAT IS HEALTH AND HEALING?

The fundamental root of our health-care crisis is the misunderstanding of health and healing. The prevailing belief in our society is, "If I feel good and I am not sick then I am healthy." This common conception of health limits people's ability to reach their optimum potential. It restricts them to a condition in which there is merely a lack of symptoms and it promotes the idea that the body should function "normal," in other words, *average*.

The current determinant of health advocated by the allopathic or medical model is an assortment of lab values and diagnostic criteria that must remain at "normal" levels based upon statistical studies of the average person. Based on the mentality of mediocrity, values such as blood pressure, cholesterol counts, hormonal levels and other data are determined through laboratory and diagnostic procedures and then compared to the levels of the average John or Jane Doe on the street. As long as these values are within a certain "allowable" range variant of these levels, you are considered healthy. If, however, these values are too high or too low, you are deemed unhealthy or "sick," and a variety of procedures can then be employed to bring you back to normal or average, using potions, lotions, pills or in more severe cases, radiation and surgery.

Our entire health-care system is based on the allopathic model of medicine. This system is founded upon a mechanistic world-view developed and promoted by René Descartes and Isaac Newton. This world-view states that the universe works like a mechanical clock. The physical world is made up of parts that work together like the gears in a machine. It is predictable and manageable. If we learn to understand its parts and how they interact, we will be able to control our environment and rule the world. This represents the mentality of medical care. If we understand all the parts in the human body, and how they function together, we can then develop strategies to keep it healthy. This is the "Curing" paradigm. Diagnosis – Treat – Cure. It is the understanding that our bodies can be controlled and brought to a state of "normal" or average. Currently, if something is too high, we lower it; if it is too low, we raise it; if it is too long, we shorten it; if it is too short, we lengthen it. When it becomes painful, we numb it, should it become numb, we stimulate it. If it becomes hard, we soften it. If it becomes too soft, we harden it. If it becomes too full, we empty it. And, if it becomes too empty, we fill it. When all has been tried and our patience (and patients) has been exhausted, we remove it.

What this "Curing" paradigm lacks is the one quality that a living body possesses that the non-living mechanical world does not: Life. There is a vital force that is inherent in all living things. This élan vital gives to our bodies that "special something" that allows us to grow under stress, experience feelings and innately heal. This life energy is unpredictable and unmanageable, yet, it is infinitely intelligent and uniquely efficient. It is an organizing and ever-evolving force, that cannot be controlled and directed through the use of pills, potions and lotions, and it is ever-seeking to be more organized, more efficient and more intelligent. This is the basis of Vitalism – the foundation of the healing model outlined in *A Clear Path to Healing*.

The basis of the allopathic or medical model is Mechanism, in which the body is viewed as a machine where parts are parts and if anything is out of the ordinary, these parts may be altered through chemistry or surgery – replaced or removed.

Whereas this approach is very effective for emergency, life or death situations, it does not promote health. The purpose of medical care is to fight disease once diagnosed, and prevent death at all costs. What lacks in this model is the concept of *disease prevention* and *health promotion*. Our current model has created a "don't fix it till it's broke" mentality. Just like an ambulance sitting at the bottom of a cliff waiting for people to jump, the medical model fails to provide a healthy quality of life for its recipients, because the person must get sick before the physician can take action.

The true key to health is *prevention* and *responsibility*. According to the World Health Organization, Japan is the healthiest country in the world.[5] Why? Their entire health-care system is based on prevention. The doctors are paid to keep you healthy through prevention and education, rather than waiting until you get sick to treat the disease.

When we speak of "healing," we address a process that is much more than the mere removal of symptoms, and when we look for "health," we seek something much more than average.

According to *Dorland's Medical Dictionary*, health is "a state of complete physical, emotional, mental, social and spiritual well-being, and not merely the absence of disease and infirmity."[6] Health is the experience of the fullest expression of ourselves and our inner gifts, talents and abilities. Health is when all our individual cells are peacefully and joyously functioning in harmony. When all our organs, tissues, glands and blood vessels are working together as a team, we have complete health.

Healing is when a part of us, that was separated, shamed, or harmed, becomes reconnected and loved. Healing is the process of becoming whole; of becoming better, stronger, and wiser. When we can look at the world with more joy, peace, and love, we have experienced healing.

The fundamental root of our health-care crisis is not escalating costs, poor insurance coverage or even the rising prevalence of disease. It is an over-emphasis on "curing" versus "healing." Our current health-care model is based on the superficial removal of symptoms bringing individuals to average health, instead of providing an improved quality of life and empowering individuals to be a greater expression of who they are, bringing them increased levels of joy, peace and freedom.

As you journey through this book, you'll explore many aspects of health and healing. You will discover deep universal truths and practical ways to apply them. I will show you how to use your mind and emotions to enhance your healing experience, as well as how to better nurture and care for your body.

Our bodies have been created in such a fashion, that if cared for properly, they will function and heal easily and effortlessly. We need not struggle to experience perfect health or suffer in reaching our optimum potential. Just as a flower effortlessly releases its scent, and our planet gracefully swims around the sun, so should the expression of who you are, freely and easily radiate from within.

1. "AMA: U.S. Health System must be fixed", December 17, 1998, CNN Interactive, CNN.com.
2. "National Health Care Expenditures", Health Care Financing Administration, www.hcfa.gov/stats/stats.htm
3. The Robert Wood Johnson Foundation, Chronic Care in America: A 21st Century Challenge; Health, United States, 1996.
4. "Japanese have longest healthy lives", USA Today, June 4, 2000.
5. ibid.
6. Dorland's Medical Dictionary, W.B. Saunders Company, Philadelphia, 1989

The Definition of Success

To laugh often and much.

To win the respect of people and the affection of children.

To earn the appreciation of honest critics

and endure the betrayal of false friends.

To appreciate beauty.

To find the best in others.

To have the world a little bit better

whether by garden patch, a healthy child,

or a redeemed social condition.

To know even one life has breathed easier because you have lived.

This is to have succeeded.

~ Ralph Waldo Emerson

2

THE BENEFITS OF ...
A Clear Path to Healing

Be the change you wish to see in others.

~ Gandhi

My mission in writing this book is to provide an easy-to-understand and easy-to-follow path for any individual to reclaim the inner healing-power which they possess. I outline a proven method to achieve whatever it is you seek in your life. Having worked with thousands of people, I discovered that when you remove the "should's" of desire, we are all searching for the same thing: A more joyful, peaceful, love-filled and freer experience of life, and a fuller expression of who we are and the unique gifts we each have to offer the world.

On your journey along a clear path to healing, you will explore timeless, universal principles to reclaim individual healing power. You will examine belief systems that inhibit you from experiencing our fullest health potential. And you will discover new tools for the mind and body that will empower you to accept responsibility for your own life and your own health.

The actions you will learn are easy and effortless in and of themselves, yet sometimes it will seem difficult to keep on the path. Life may catch up to you and you may forget or neglect to do what is necessary in order to stay on this journey. To stay focused you must have a clear picture of why you are doing this. In chapter 8, Think and Grow Healthy, you will learn techniques to create and maintain a vision of health and wellness.

Quite often we do not want to eat right, meditate or exercise, however, if we focus on the benefits that these actions bring us, we can inspire ourselves to take action and move forward.

On the following pages are the most profound benefits you will experience while on this path to healing. These benefits are divided into two categories: the benefits to you as an individual living by the principles and practices in this book; and the benefits to the world, if everyone began to walk a clear path to healing.

INDIVIDUAL BENEFITS

Clarity and Peace of Mind

Understand the principles of healing and you will begin to see the world in a new way. Much of your confusion and anxiety will fall away and a new clarity and an experience of peacefulness will begin to fill your mind. Often it is the disempowering and false beliefs that create the veil that covers your eyes to the joy and wisdom that is available to you. When the veil is lifted you are able to see with clear vision, the world as a much brighter place, where chaos and distortion are replaced with meaning and light.

Follow the principles and practices of healing, and your body will begin to shed old toxins and tension that interfere with clear thought. The mind can become cluttered with negativity and distraction due to the "garbage in the field." When you begin to clean your body by eating healthy food, drinking clean water, taking deep breaths, exercising, and getting adequate rest, a clarity of thought begins to develop in your mind and you begin to feel much more peaceful and calm.

Experiencing this clarity and peace of mind, makes it much easier to stay on this clear path to healing and you will benefit with a healthier, more fulfilling life.

Increased Adaptability to Stress

In chapter 6, The Seven Attributes of Health, you will learn it is not stress that causes disease, but the inability to respond appropriately that is the culprit. On the clear path to healing, your body and mind becomes more sensitive to the environment, and becomes more aware of subtle changes that, in the past, may have been invisible to you. Along with this increased perception, you become much more efficient and effective at adapting to these changes. Using less energy and more coordination, what was once stressful, is now joyful, and things that troubled you pass over your shoulders like a gentle breeze.

Increased Energy and Vitality

Increased energy and vitality are two benefits on the clear path to healing. As the mind becomes clearer and the body cleaner, you experience more strength and power. Renewed energy will drive you forward to be more, do more and achieve more. Every day as you clarify your vision of health, you feel more alive, as if the energy is emerging from an endless pool deep within the core of your being. The more energy you express, the more you will be blessed with an infinite supply of energy and vitality.

Greater Strength, Confidence, and Personal Power

Through the mental and physical exercises presented in this book, both your mental faculties and physical health will begin to grow in strength. Like a muscle that grows under weight, your entire being will begin to strengthen and become more powerful. As you grow stronger, you will see that you are capable of many great things. With this awareness, you will appreciate yourself more and an empowering confidence will fill you. With each accomplishment along the way, your personal power will become more evident and more present. This growing strength, confidence and power makes it easier to stay on your healing path, and your physical and mental energies begin to focus on bigger and grander avenues of creativity, contribution and purpose.

Increased Wisdom and Knowledge

With a clearer and more peaceful mind, and a stronger, more powerful body, you will step out into the world with a new point of view. A veil of illusion will lift from your eyes. Things that didn't make sense in the past, you now understand, and what you were unaware of, now appears commonplace.

On a clear path to healing, it is common for people to spontaneously become more in tune to things that alluded them before. With this increased awareness and clarity of mind, you begin to understand the world in ways that you would have never thought of before. With this knowledge and understanding, you develop wisdom. Through this wisdom you are able to make better choices and discover new things about yourself and the world around you.

Improved Relationships with Others

As you continue to understand yourself, you understand others as well. When you experience that we are all one, you will begin to treat others as you treat yourself. Every great spiritual master has taught us, that we are each other's keeper and not only are we responsible for ourselves, but also accountable to others. By practicing this in your daily life, your heart will open to greater levels of love, communication and companionship and your interactions with your friends, loved ones, business partners and community neighbors will begin to miraculously blossom into harmonious, healthy, supportive, and loving relationships.

Increased Creativity, Prosperity and Spontaneous Manifestation of Goals and Dreams

I consider this to be the most exciting and rewarding, but not the last benefit, that you achieve on this healing path. When you strengthen your body and mind through the learned practices, you experience an increased manifestation of your dreams and desires. Things that once seemed the fancy of an imaginative dreamer, will become real in your life. The ability to create in physical form your emotional and mental imaginings increases, and your life of struggle, lack and failure is replaced with a life of effortless ease, abundant prosperity and unlimited success. By staying focused on your vision and veering not to the left or right of this path, each day becomes a blessing, and every stepping stone a *Garden of Eden*, a Heaven on Earth of your own creation.

GLOBAL BENEFITS

When we heal ourselves, we heal the world. Every action we take to improve our own life, we set a cause in motion improving the lives of everyone we meet. With every harmonious interaction you have with others, you influence them to take responsibility for their lives, and like a domino that touches the next, a stream of health begins to flow throughout our communities and out into the world. This is the true clear path to healing.

One person walking this path, shows a thousand more the way. As a tiny flame sparks an enormous blaze, so too, can this wave of healing wash away disease, hardship and despair and let us live together as one family on this earth, just as it was meant to be from the beginning.

Let's take a moment to look at some of the important benefits that as a society, we can delight in if each of us acts locally within ourselves, but thinks globally ... for with each action and thought we take to improve ourselves, we contribute to a happier, healthier world.

Less Mental Illness and Addiction

As each of us begins to experience a clearer and more peaceful mind, depression, anxiety and other mental illnesses that plague our societies will slowly vanish. With the love and support of other people, and our growing ability to handle stress, events and circumstances that cause us grief no longer occur, or are presented to us as opportunities for growth and learning. In time, as our minds become healthier and our lives more fulfilling, the desire to escape from reality will become less. The joy and fulfillment of achieving our most endearing dreams and intentions, overcomes the need for the numbing effects of alcohol, drugs, and other addictive behaviors. Addictions become choices, and what bound us in chains loses its power over us.

Stress-free Society

The universe and everything within it is in a constant state of change. Because of this, our lives are never free from the influence of stress. However, by strengthening our bodies and minds, and increasing our ability to respond peacefully and effectively to these changes, we will not be overwhelmed by its presence. Change in the environment will "blow through our leaves" easily and effortlessly allowing us to grow, learn and evolve from each experience. Free from the negative effects of stress overload, we will focus our lives on the accomplishment of great deeds and meaningful purpose.

Environmental Purity

Keeping our bodies clean and our minds clear and focused, our actions in the outside world work in harmony with our planet. With each of us intent on giving our gifts and sharing our love through harmonious interactions, we are prevented from doing anything that would damage our Mother Earth. On this clear path to healing, not only will our bodies and minds become healthier, but our rivers, streams, lakes and oceans will become cleaner. Our soil will be more rich and our air cleaner to breathe. The plants and animals that we have been entrusted to nurture and protect, will become our friends and not run from our presence. Only by cleaning the environment within us, will we enjoy the benefits of a clean environment outside of us. Having achieved this, a harmonious interaction between ourselves and the Earth will develop, both mutually supportive of creating our Garden of Eden.

Less Physical Disease

As more people become responsible for their own lives – keeping their bodies clean of toxins and more adaptable to stress – things that once caused internal disease will cause the body to become stronger and more evolved. Disease and illness that plague our society won't be present, because people will be resistant to such influences. Every individual who keeps themselves healthy through prevention, positive thought and nourishing behaviors, causes disease to pass from consciousness into the realm of illusion, never to be seen again.

Scientific and Technological Advancement

Understanding the universal principles that govern creation, and achieving more subtle levels of awareness and higher planes of knowledge and wisdom, our advances in science and technology will eclipse what we have today, making our current cutting-edge research and development appear as the discovery of fire and the carving of the first spear. Our technology will allow us to travel to distant stars, possibly in the vehicle of our own bodies, and allow us to utilize energy and power from the essence of the very space around us. What we now consider science fiction, will become common place and what we will be capable of, sits at the furthest reaches of our imagination. Most importantly, this technology will no longer be of a damaging and destructive nature or create further problems such as endangered species, toxic environments and increased disease and suffering. Our endeavors to expand our awareness and knowledge, and to progress our science and technology will create further opportunities for our evolution and advancement and simplify our lives without creating problems that are to complex to solve.

International Peace and Elimination of Criminal Activity

Knowing that we create our own reality and that we are all one energy, the desire to hurt or harm will no longer exist. Just like the conditions of our body and mind that disappeared, so will the diseases of our society vanish from our world. Crime, war and expressions of hate will no longer plague our society. International peace will wash across this planet in a vast wave of cleansing love, and we will witness crime vanish from our city streets as communities of healthy, fulfilled individuals grow. Expressions and actions of hate and competition won't be present in our lives, because we will learn that there is an infinite source for all and that there is nothing that we can't have, nothing we can't do and nothing we can't be.

Increased Prosperity for All

Have you noticed that we live in a creative universe? Anything we imagine, we can create in our lives. In fact, the only way you can experience a specific desire or intention is if you have the ability to attain it.

You are a powerful, creative being. You have gifts and abilities yet to discover. As a result of your journey, you will approach your fullest potential and your dearest desire. The universe in its abundance lacks nothing. All that you hold dear in your heart can be yours if you remain true to yourself and witness the principles in action by following the practices found herein.

There is prosperity for all. There is no need to compete or to fight. We create through the positive power of our body and mind.

I sense your anticipation and excitement to set foot on this journey to healing. I imagine the determination in your eyes and the enthusiasm in your voice. However, before you begin, it is important that you make yourself aware of what has inhibited you from optimum health and healing in the past. As my grandmother used to say, "We gotta clean out the bad, before we can put in the good."

The first step will be to take a look at "The Beaten Path" of the outworn, "curing" model. When we understand what caused this crisis of health-care from the onset, we can then work to change it.

In the following two chapters, we'll explore the seven fundamental causes of the health-care crisis, as well as the seven false beliefs, or illusions, which inhibit health and healing. I have also outlined seven new beliefs or principles that you can begin to incorporate into your life, to assist you to take your first steps toward a whole new world of peace, joy and health.

Let us begin our journey on *A Clear Path to Healing*.

PART I

THE BEATEN PATH

3

EXPOSING THE CRISIS

The doctor of the future will give no medicine, but will interest his patients in the care of the human frame, in diet, and in the cause and prevention of disease. ~ *Thomas Edison*

First, do no harm. ~ *Florence Nightingale*

As both a member of the health-care industry and a recipient of its services, I have found that there are seven fundamental causes creating the present health-care crisis. These seven causes have not been created by specific individuals, institutions or doctrines, but by all collectively – imbedded in our culture and our way of thinking. The state of our health-care system and our community's current level of health is nothing more than a reflection of deeper cultural and personal issues – societal mores entrained into our minds and reinforced by our belief systems.

However easy it is to point fingers and throw blame at the powers that be, if we are to truly discover what inhibits us from our fullest expression of health and healing, we must look at ourselves and the deeper issues that are the true cause.

In this chapter, we will examine each of the seven causes in depth. Although I may confront the doctrines and methods of a few traditional health-care institutions, and challenge their beliefs, principles and intentions, I do this not to pass judgment nor to blame, but to shed light upon a possible danger to the health of our community.

Every effect has a specific cause. If we are to experience complete healing, whether on a personal or a community level, we must find the cause and change it.

The current health-care crisis is a "dis-ease" that exists on an individual, cultural and societal level. To heal this crisis, we must be honest and open-minded, allowing us to look within ourselves, our establishments, and our society, and examine them for possible causes. When we find something that is not in our best interest, which interferes with our ability to live to our fullest potential, we then can accept the possibility that our thoughts and actions, up to this point, have not been effective. With this awareness and acknowledgment, we can make the change.

As you take the first steps on your clear path to healing, you will find that the path might not be clear. The path will be thick and dense, obscured by the underbrush of belief systems, past actions, and a fearful heart. Beyond this untamed wild of bracken and thicket, lies the clear healing path we seek. If we are to reach our destination we must first eliminate that which holds us back.

The clear path to healing is not something that I can give to you. It lies dormant within each one of us, waiting to be released. By examining yourself, as well as the institutions and doctrines you support, by being open to change, you can break through the barriers that are holding you back from optimum health and well-being.

Let's now look at those things that have created the health-care crisis (whether personal or societal) we are now experiencing.

CAUSE #1

Lack of Responsibility

Often when we hear the word "responsibility" we cringe because it brings forth images of work, obligation and limitation. For some it causes feelings of guilt, shame or resentment. Before you slam the book down with the mere mention of the word, let me define "responsibility." When you understand this word, it becomes a vehicle through which you achieve joy, power, and inner strength.

When I use the word responsibility I define two things: *responsibility* and *response ability*. *Responsibility* is the ability to consciously choose behaviors that are in the best interest of yourself and others, and to act upon those choices. *Response ability* is the ability to respond appropriately to the changes in our internal and external environment – consciously or sub-consciously.

Our ability to respond to the world around us and make appropriate and empowering decisions, will allow us to be healthy and to reach our optimum potential both as individuals and as a community. Understanding this, we choose to seek our highest expression of responsibility, rather than cower at its mere mention.

Lack of responsibility is the first cause of the current health-care crisis. Because of this lack, more and more people are getting sicker while spending more money on health-care.

Health and healing can be quite automatic and effortless, however, there are certain responsibilities that must be acted upon by the individual. Certain things must be maintained through responsible action.

When you buy a car, it takes only the turn of the key and a push on the accelerator to make it go. However, if you do not maintain the car, eventually it breaks down and no longer serves you. If you do not put in gasoline and oil, change the spark plugs, rotate the tires, and clean and wax the outside, in time, the car will decay and fall apart. If we accept responsibility and take the appropriate actions, a car that might last five years without maintenance, may last fifty years with care, and become a valuable classic.

The same holds true for our bodies. There are certain actions we need to take – which are easy and effortless – in order for us to live a healthy, vibrant life. We must fuel our bodies with clean, nutrient rich foods. We must exercise our bodies, keeping them strong and long-lasting. We must take in adequate amounts of water and air, receive adequate rest, and avoid putting things into our bodies that will cause it to decay or malfunction. Like the car, it is up to us to accept responsibility for our actions, if we are to expect and appreciate a healthy, long-lasting body.

When we look at the most common diseases and the leading causes of death in our country, we see a very familiar list: cancer, heart disease, stroke and diabetes. What do these conditions all have in common? They are all preventable and are often the result of a lack of responsibility over the course of many years, sometimes even decades. These common, and often fatal conditions are usually the result of neglect and indifference. If you look at the history of the sufferers of these ailments you will commonly see years of poor diet, little or no exercise, negative thinking and possibly an overuse of alcohol, cigarettes, processed foods, and pharmaceutical and recreational drugs.

Unfortunately, the degenerative effects of these habits take years to demonstrate their disease-causing effects. By the time the individual is aware of the consequence of their actions, the damage has already been done, and they find themselves in a state of crisis. Unable to make the necessary changes to reverse the damaging effects they must run to the doctor, who will accept responsibility for them and give them medicine to "fix" them.

However, they are never "fixed." Instead, they are brought to a state of average, using whatever chemical and surgical means is necessary, with no improvement of their quality of life. Without the education to learn how to take responsibility for themselves, they continue their careless habits, addictions and behaviors, and sit day in and day out in a recliner in front of the television set in some assisted living-facility allowing their bodies and minds to decay before their very eyes.

Millions of dollars are spent every week on senior citizens such as these, with the sole purpose to keep them alive without any improvement in the quality of their life. These dollars are provided from other citizens – to those who can no longer accept responsibility for themselves – in the form of taxes. This is a contradiction in that, those who are taking responsibility for themselves, are penalized by having to provide the financial resources to keep those who do not, barely alive.

It is my intention to provide you with information for you to accept responsibility for your own life and your own health. As stated earlier, *"if you give a man a fish, you feed him for a day, but if you teach him how to fish, you feed him for a lifetime."* The purpose of this book is to teach you how to accept responsibility for your life and to live to your fullest potential, full of vitality and with a zest for life, even at advanced ages, rather than becoming another nursing-home patron, dependent on tax dollars, social security and medicare to keep you barely alive with a bare minimum quality of life.

Whereas accepting responsibility is the first and most important step on the clear path to healing, our body and mind's "Response Ability" is also vital in addressing the issues of health and healing. Response ability is our body and mind's innate ability to respond appropriately and efficiently to changes and stresses within our immediate environment.

As another cause of our health-care crisis, the weakening or loss of our Response Ability is what I have come to understand to be the cause of all disease, which will be discussed in chapters 6 and 7. This understanding is key to achieving optimum health and well-being. The greater our ability to handle change and stress in our environment, the greater our experience of optimum health and vitality.

CAUSE #2

Encouraged Apathy

The second cause of our current health-care crisis is an overall attitude amongst our society of not caring. Today, more than ever, the concern of most is to get just enough education to make just enough money to pay the bills and get just enough food on the table and clothes on their backs. Even with the current knowledge and understanding of disease prevention in regards to diet, exercise, spinal care and other health issues, people still walk around with the attitude, "If it ain't broke, don't fix it."

What is worse than the *apathy* itself is that this attitude is supported, and even encouraged, by pharmaceutical companies, health maintenance organizations, and other health-care providers. These organizations feed off the disease and illnesses of others. It is only through the misfortune of individuals such as you and I, that these institutions can even exist. For if we were empowered to accept responsibility for ourselves and to take action to improve our quality of life, they would have nothing to offer us in the way of product or service.

Imagine what would happen to these institutions if suddenly everyone took responsibility for their health and ate well-balanced, healthy meals, exercised, and eliminated cigarettes, alcohol and drugs. These institutions would either reconstruct themselves to provide for these consumers or they would collapse.

To begin to resolve our health-care crisis, we must take individual initiative to educate ourselves and then take responsibility to act on what we have learned. Only by removing *apathy* through careful attention and passionate regard, will we free ourselves from the bondage of disease and live to our fullest potential.

CAUSE #3

Unwavering Traditionalism

The third cause of our health-care crisis is what I call *Unwavering Traditionalism*. This is our society's tendency to find comfort in their agreed-upon world-view and cultural belief system, regardless of how untrue, disempowering or outdated it may be.

Once someone discovers a belief system that seems to work for them, holding them in a state of mediocrity or "normal," it is very difficult to have them change, regardless of how ludicrous and ridiculous the belief system is. Being resistant and reluctant to change these beliefs, they continue to live in a world which no longer exists or ever existed. Our history is filled with examples of people living in a world of illusion created by the veil of their own beliefs.

For thousands of years it was believed that the world was flat and that the Earth was the center of the universe, with the sun, planets and stars orbiting its regal fortress. When the great astronomer Copernicus announced that the Earth orbited the sun, and was in fact just another body amongst an infinite cosmic sea of stars, planets and galaxies, he was declared a heretic. Copernicus himself states that "...the scorn which I had to fear on account of the newness and absurdity of my opinion almost drove me to abandon a work already undertaken."[1]

When one-hundred years later, Galileo invented the telescope and confirmed Copernicus' ideas, he was severely persecuted and placed under a treacherous ordeal of prison, trials and near-assassination, forcing him to abandon his "foolishness."

Look at this declaration from Pope Urban VII and the Lord Cardinal Inquisitors of the Roman Catholic Church accusing Galileo of heresy for announcing publicly that the Earth is not the center of the universe and revolves around the sun:

> "We ... sentence, and declare that you, the said Galileo, by reasons brought forth in trial, and by you confessed as above, have rendered yourself in the judgment of this Holy Office vehemently suspected of heresy, namely, of having believed and held the doctrine which is false and contrary to the Sacred and Divine Scriptures, that the sun is the center of the world and does not move from east to west and that the Earth moves and is not the center of the world ...

> " ...and you may be absolved (of these crimes), provided that, first ... you abjure, curse and detest before us the aforesaid errors and heresies and every other error and heresy contrary to the Catholic and Apostolic Roman Church in the form to be prescribed by us for you."

Humiliated and broken by the pressure of the Church and threat of torture, Galileo responded in 1633:

"I, Galileo ... aged seventy years, arraigned personally before this tribunal and kneeling before you, Most Eminent and Lord Cardinals Inquisitors General against heretical pravity throughout the entire Christian Commonwealth ... I ... abandon the false opinion that the Earth is not the center of the world and moves ... and I abjure, curse and detest the aforesaid errors and heresies contrary to the Holy Church...and I promise to carry out ... all penances that have been or shall be imposed upon me by this Holy Office..."[2]

Shortly after, the Church received tremendous pressure from its subjects, and continual confirmation by other scientists forced the Pope to accept the ideas of both Copernicus and Galileo. After this incident, the Church was careful about opposing the findings of the scientific community.

Christopher Columbus was initially laughed at and ridiculed when he returned to Spain with the discovery that the world is round. In fact, Queen Isabella of Spain, after seven years of petitions, allowed Columbus only to take prisoners on his journey, for she "knew" they would fall off the edge of the Earth anyway.[3]

The concepts of manned flight, horse-less carriages, electric lighting, radio, television, and personal computers were all scoffed at and considered at one time to be mere fantasies of a delusional mind. For Lord Kelvin said in 1897, "Radio has no future," and in 1898, Charles H. Duell, commissioner of the U.S. Patent Office said that they might as well close up shop, for everything that could possibly be invented had been.[4]

All new ideas, philosophies and creative innovations generally move through four stages. First, they are laughed at and ridiculed. Second, they are considered possibilities. Third, they are accepted as fact, and lastly, and quite humorously, the general public claims it as their own, often expressing their satisfaction of "knowing it all along" or actually of having discovered the idea themselves.

We are currently experiencing a similar situation in the realm of health-care. The most dramatic is the concept of the Germ Theory. For the last one-hundred years, based upon the research of Louis Pasteur, it has been believed that the germ – the bacteria, virus or toxin – is the cause of disease. What is not readily accepted and acknowledged is the brief realization Louis expressed on his death-bed. What has been overlooked and ignored to this day are his last words as he died. Translated from the original French, Pasteur said, "It is not the germ ... it's the soil."[5] These words changed the substance of his research, yet the false premise of the Germ Theory is still the dominating model of health-care. According to his last words, the bacteria and viruses could no longer be looked upon as the cause of disease. The cause of disease is in the "soil." The bacteria and viruses are mere opportunists which find a safe home and feed off an already weakened body. Let me explain with a story.

One day, a cow was walking through a beautiful pasture. Beneath a bright blue, sunny sky, the cow peacefully grazed on the green grass. Nothing disturbed her silent repose. Suddenly, the cow lifted her tail and relieved herself, creating an impressive pile of manure in the center of the field. Turning her head to examine her masterpiece, she gave a nod and lifted her chin, and continued her morning walk, grazing in bliss. As she walked away into the distance, a swarm of flies began to gather around the manure, delighting in the delicacy provided by the cow. The moral of the story is one's waste is another's treasure.

You are probably wondering why I just told this story. Besides adding a little comic relief it was to pose a pertinent question: Are the flies the problem? Are the flies the cause of the mess? Obviously, the answer is No. You can swat the flies all you want, use chemical repellents, even light it on fire … if the field is not cleaned of manure, you will always have flies. Why then do we use antibiotics, vaccinations and other drugs to fight off germs? Are we not swatting flies? We are attacking the germs without cleaning up the mess.

In order to achieve optimum health and vitality, we must accept the responsibility to stop swatting the flies, and begin to strengthen the body and "clean up the field."

Our bodies have a remarkable system for removing the "garbage from the field." It is called the immune system. The cells that make up this system migrate around the body removing bacteria, viruses, toxins and other foreign objects from the body, keeping the field clean. It is not the germs that cause the disease, but a breakdown in the proper functioning of the immune system.

You will learn further along your path to healing, strategies to increase your response ability so that these tiny opportunistic varmints no longer find your body a safe and beneficial place to be.

A Word on Vaccinations

One of the greatest blunders currently being imposed upon the human community is that of vaccinations. Vaccinations were presented to our communities as a means by which our children could be protected from the dangerous effects of disease. The theory states that by injecting minute doses of the actual disease into our body, our body would innately produce antibodies or immune factors to protect itself from the vaccine, developing an immunity and protecting the individual from future exposure to the disease. At some point in the past, the scientific knowledge of the day confirmed the truth of vaccinations. However, as our scientific understanding has expanded, we now know that vaccines are a false premise. Yet, even though we know they are no longer valid, the scientific and medical community still hold to their belief of vaccinations, just as the Church held onto the notion of an earth-centered universe.

Even if this theory did hold true, what has been found is that the promoted benefit of vaccines does not substantiate their unpublished risks. Before we examine the dangers of vaccines, let's first look at the evidence of their fallacy. According to the eye-opening book, *Immunization: The Reality Behind the Myth* by Walene James, all diseases have cycles of virulence and dormancy.[6] Let us take polio, for example.

In 1920, the death rate of the polio virus had begun a steady decline. In fact, by 1940, the incidence of polio had decreased 50%. When the polio vaccines had been introduced between 1953 and 1959, the death rate of polio had already reduced between 75 and 80% naturally by itself.[7] The disease had been on its way out when the developers of the vaccine declared themselves the heroes. Since 1980, the only incidences of polio have been caused by the vaccine.[8]

In *Vaccines: Are They Really Safe and Effective*, by Dr. Harris Coulter, similar scenarios are evident with all other vaccines. The death rate of Pertussis (the 'P' in DPT), also called whooping cough, decreased more than 75% before the vaccine was introduced. The measles death rate reduced more than 95% before the vaccine was introduced.[9] If the vaccine was truly the cause of the reduction of this disease, wouldn't the drug have been introduced before the reduction in the death rate?

When we examine the detrimental effects that vaccines have on our children, it arouses feelings of anger and concern. According to Cynthia Cournoyer, in her book, *What about Immunization? Exposing the Vaccine Philosophy*, the following statistics brought tears to my eyes:

Rates of Reactions Per Year in the U.S.
of Children Vaccinated with DPT

1 in 20:	Persistent Crying
1 in 66:	High Fever
1 in 180:	High Pitched Screaming
1 in 350:	Convulsions
1 in 350:	Shock or Collapse
1 in 22,000:	Acute Brain Disorder
1 in 62,000:	Permanent Brain Damage
1 in 71,600:	Death

Of the last three statistics, there are over 35,000 children affected every year. Besides these children who now suffer from permanent brain damage and perhaps died, 11,000 to 12,000 other children each year begin to experience the following symptoms, sometimes a year after receiving the vaccinations: developmental delay, learning disabilities, hyperactivity, behavior disorder, autism, epilepsy and profound retardation.[10]

The book goes on to say that there is a 94 times greater risk of dying from the DPT vaccine than from the disease. There is a 3.888 times greater risk of acquiring long term damage from the vaccine than from the disease itself. It then also states, "If that does not shock you, there are about 10 deaths every year from the disease and at least 943 deaths per year from the vaccine. There are only 3 cases of long term damage from the disease per year, but at least 11,666 cases of long term damage every year from the vaccine."[11]

The following story by Amy Rosenbaum Clark was found in the September 1994 issue of *Vegetarian Times* and demonstrates the devastating effects vaccines have on children and their families.

Mikey's Story

"Less than 30 minutes after his first diptheria-pertussis-tetanus (DPT) immunization, seven-month-old Michael Daly of Oak Park, Illinois began to cry inconsolably. Over the next 24 hours, his temperature shot up to 103 degrees.

"For the four days that followed, Michael was less ill but displayed odd symptoms: his fever lessened but lingered; he could not sit or walk because his leg was hard, swollen and hot where the shot had been administered; he startled easily and screamed at normal noises; and his mother, Sharon, could not engage him in play. 'My doctor assured me that this was a severe, but *normal* reaction.' She says

"Later that week, Michael smiled for the first time in five days. When his mother went to get him out of his crib the next morning, she found him dead. 'Prior to his vaccination, I had a delightful, active and healthy boy, who at seven months was already walking while holding onto furniture.'" [12]

Although this story may shock you, you may cast it aside as a fluke or happenstance. Don't be so quick to disregard this incident for over 12,000 such incidences occur every year from the DPT shot alone.[13] This is not a chance occurrence. This is a serious risk that must be considered.

Although the risks of vaccinations are scary enough, what is even more frightening is that we do not have a choice. In all 50 states, it is mandatory for our children to be vaccinated to attend public schools, qualify for insurance, get driving licenses and even get jobs.[14] If a parent is informed of the risks and decides with an educated mind that they wish their children to be vaccinated, I bless them and respect their decision. But what of the parent who makes a different choice? What if they understand that their child has a powerful inner healer and doesn't need the poisons injected into their body to develop a healthy immune system, but also does not want to subject their child to the deadly risks of the vaccine? Must they be forced to vaccinate with the threat of an uneducatable, unemployable child? I think not. If you wish to learn more about vaccinations and learn how to protect your children from their dangers, see the resource section in the back of this book and acquire information on organizations and books that are on your side and protecting our children.

Are you beginning to see how a false and unswerving belief and worldview that is proven to be no longer true can infiltrate and dominate a societal mind? Are you beginning to realize how people support and defend these false premises, even when the creator of the idea himself invalidated it? Why do people defend such false beliefs, even when these beliefs no longer serve and may even harm them? Let's look at another example currently within our health-care system.

Another traditional belief is that our body is a machine made up of parts that can be altered, exchanged or removed. Our body is not a machine made of parts, but an intelligently organized whole working in infinite efficiency capable of growth, experience and learning. Often a doctor practicing within the allopathic – medical model will look at the person as a condition or sick part and forget that they are dealing with a live human being.

Healing is about creating wholeness, not separation. By removing a part, such as the appendix, gall bladder or tonsils, we create greater separation, which will eventually lead to more disease. By treating the part and not the person, further separation is created, and healing will never result. Although our society continues to support this scientifically disproven model regardless of the consequences, it no longer serves us. It prevents us from reaching our true potential as a human being.

Why do we continue to support and defend these beliefs? There are two reasons. First is the herd mentality, second, the fear of the unknown.

People tend to follow the masses in an effort to belong and feel loved. Often people will believe and do anything, regardless of the long-term consequences, if it means they will be accepted. One of the greatest fears we experience is the fear of rejection, a survey cited by *The Book of Lists* would have us believe. In this poll, public speaking was number one on America's fear-and-loathing hit parade, easily topping flying, snakes, loneliness and even death itself (seventh on the list).[15] Why do so many people suffer this fear? What they fear is the idea of being unaccepted, rejected and alone. They will accept anything the majority has approved, including their view of the world, if it means being a part of the herd.

The other reason for this *unwavering traditionalism* is a fear of the unknown – people do not like uncertainty. They want to know what lies ahead. If their current world-view and belief system has worked until now, why accept something new if there is the possibility of harm, or even worse, *change*. People would rather live in mediocrity and be average, providing safety and security, than to adventure into the unknown. Yet, it is only in uncertainty that growth lies. Only in what is unknown will we find the deeper truths of life, self and healing.

If we are to amend the current health-care crisis, the institutions of health-care and its recipients will need to be open to change and must adopt a new philosophic and scientific understanding.

"If you do what you've always done, you'll get what you've always gotten." ~ *Henry Ford*

CAUSE #4

Nurtured Fear

Two of the largest industries in the world are the Pharmaceutical and Insurance industries. The purpose of these industries is to provide security and comfort to people in times of crisis. Whereas these companies provide a very valuable and needed service, they also support something that not only interferes with health and healing, but promotes a major cause of disease and the crisis they claim to be protecting us from: *Fear*.

Many in our society live in a perpetual state of fear. Fear of poverty. Fear of crime. Fear of crisis. Fear of accidents. Fear of disease. This fear has fostered a multi-trillion dollar insurance industry. Individuals spend thousands of dollars every month to protect themselves just in case something happens. Insurance premiums are the highest ever because people are willing to pay to have their fears comforted. By paying a monthly or annual payment, you can rest assured that should anything occur, the insurance company will be there to protect you from financial ruin.

In this financial arena, everything can be insured with the development of car insurance, home insurance, disability insurance (in case you can't work due to injury), liability and malpractice insurance (in case some one gets hurt in your presence), health insurance and life insurance.

Understanding your insecurity and fear as the basis of their business, insurance companies nurture the fears of the public. Promoting images of illness, injury, catastrophe, financial ruin and death, they trigger the deepest anxieties in consumers, who then run to them for security and peace of mind. Although insurance is excellent protection in the case of an emergency, the way it is promoted and purchased is another contributing factor of the health-care crisis. When people live in fear, and when their fears are continually being nurtured, you have a society that inevitably experiences the things they are trying to protect themselves from.

Pharmaceutical companies also nurture fear. There is such dread of symptoms and disease that over-the-counter drugs accounted for more than 132 billion dollars spent last year alone, to help people rid themselves of these uncomfortable experiences.[16] Afraid that discomfort and symptoms lead to disease and death, people do what they can, to rid themselves of them. Every year, the average American watches 30,000 television ads and newsreels that show them how to do just that. This is sponsored by the drug companies.[17]

Do you see how these businesses foster fear and disease? Why would a drug company cure a disease, when that very disease makes them billions of dollars? Why would an insurance company promote individual power, when that level of security would dismiss the need for insurance?

They wouldn't. In fact, they spend billions of dollars a year on marketing and advertising to make sure the level of fear and disease in this country will sustain their profit margin. Do you see the contradiction? Can you understand why both health costs and disease rates are going up? It appears that while the drug and insurance conglomerates present themselves as the solution to the health-care dilemma, they are actually a part of its cause.

Healing can not occur in a state of fear. According to Dr. Candice Pert, in her book, *Molecules of Emotion*, emotional states of fear, depression, and adverse stress create chemical and hormonal changes in our body that cause accelerated aging and degeneration.[18] These changes put our body and mind in a state of protection and alarm – fight or flight. These hormonal and biochemical conditions are diametrically opposite to those that occur during healing, repair, and growth. In this state of fear, it is physiologically impossible to heal and grow. Fear is the greatest inhibitor of health and the foremost deterrent of reaching our fullest potential and expression of who we are.

Once you learn the principles of healing and begin implementing the strategies herein, you will come to realize that there is nothing to fear, and that security comes not from insurance or drugs, but from the innate power within you.

CAUSE #5

Objective Dogma

There is a popular opinion that unless something can be objectively proven with time-tested, clinical double-blind studies based on the scientific method then it is not true. The whole notion of a unique, individual inner experience or the possibility of an integrative spiritual component of our world is labeled ludicrous without objective "proof." The only thing that is true, is that which is validated by this method of calculated scrutiny, and anything revealed or experienced in any other way is chastised as quackery, fantasy, or mental illness. I have called this notion *Objective Dogma*.

There are a number of problems with this concept. The first and most poignant is the fact that the most brilliant minds in science achieved their greatest discoveries and achievements in a single moment of inspiration and spiritual catharsis. It is through what Joseph Chilton Pierce called "The Crack in the Cosmic Egg" in that all new thought emerges to bring forth innovation and discovery. This *Eureka!* experience happened to Albert Einstein while in silent prayer he realized the basis of his Relativity Theory. Most, if not all, scientific discoveries happen in a flash of inspiration. Only later, after many years of investigation, do we understand its implication.[19]

More disturbing is the second problem caused by Objective Dogma. Although medical science claims that their procedures, pharmaceuticals, and protocols are methodically and objectively confirmed, it has been shown in the article, "Where is the Wisdom...?," by Dr. David Eddy in the esteemed *British Medical Journal* that "...only about 15% of medical interventions are supported by scientific evidence... This is partly because only 1% of the articles in medical journals are scientifically sound."[20] Why would the medical arena make such a fuss about scientific proof, when only 15% of their procedures are scientifically supported and 1% of their peer-reviewed articles are scientifically sound? Is it any wonder why 106,000 people died last year from ill effects of "properly" prescribed drugs?[21,22]

According to Dr. Barbara Starfield, MD, MPH, in her article "Is US Health Really the Best in the World," found in the July 26, 2000 issue of the *Journal of the American Medical Association*, she states:

"The health care system also may contribute to poor health through its adverse affects. For example U.S. estimates of the combined effect or errors and adverse effects that occur because of iatrogenic, or doctor caused, damage not associated with recognizable error include:

- 12,000 deaths per year from unnecessary surgery
- 7,000 deaths per year from medication errors in hospitals
- 20,000 deaths per year from other errors in hospitals
- 80,000 deaths per year from nosocomial (originated in hospital) infections in hospitals
- 106,000 deaths per year from nonerror, adverse effects of medication.

These total to 225,000 deaths per year from iatrogenic causes. Three caveats should be noted. First most of the data are derived from studies in hospitalized patients. Second, these estimates are for deaths only and do not include adverse effects that are associated with disability or discomfort.

Third, the estimates due to error are lower than those in the *Institute of Medicine Report*. If the higher estimates are used, the deaths due to iatrogenic causes would range from 230,000 to 284,000. In any case, 225,000 deaths per year constitute the Third Leading Cause of Death in the United States, after deaths from heart disease and cancer!"[22]

Every day in newspapers and journals across the country you find articles reporting medical procedures which are supposed to be scientifically secure, yet are still a guessing game – extremely dangerous and uncertain. According to Dr. Lucian Leape, in his article "Error in Medicine" found in the December 21, 1994 issue of the *Journal of the American Medical Association*, "For years, medical and nursing students have been taught Florence Nightingale's dictum – *first, do no harm*. Yet, evidence from a number of sources, reported over several decades, indicates that a substantial number of patients suffer iatrogenic, or treatment-caused, injuries while in the hospital.

"In 1964, Schimmel reported that 20% of patients admitted to a university hospital medical service suffered iatrogenic injury and that 20% of those injuries were serious or fatal. Steel, et al, found that 36% of patients admitted to a university medical service in a teaching hospital suffered an iatrogenic event of 25% were serious or life threatening. More than half of those injuries were related to medication. In 1991, Bedell et al reported the results of an analysis of cardiac arrests at a teaching hospital. They found that 64% were preventable. Again, inappropriate use of drugs were the cause of the cardiac arrests.

"If these rates are typical of the United States, then 180,000 people die each year partly as a result of iatrogenic injury, the equivalent of three jumbo-jet crashes every 2 days."[23]

In providing the following examples from newspapers around the country, my intention is not to ridicule or bad-mouth medicine or doctors. Doctors of medicine are valuable leaders in our community who can save us in times of crisis. Even though their expertise is vital for the well-being of our community, saving lives and prolonging the lives of the chronically ill, their technology and procedures are dangerous and should be approached with caution. These methods of treatment are strictly for fighting disease and trauma, they are not for preventing disease and promoting health.

Take a look at these headlines that appeared in newspapers across the country in the last few years:

"Last Year, 250,000 back surgeries were performed. Less than 10% were necessary." – *San Francisco Spine Institute* [24]

"Human error clouds results of mammograms. Radiologists often disagree on how to interpret the results of a woman's mammogram."
– *New England Journal of Medicine* [25]

"Removing wrong lung will cost hospital $5 million."
– *Associated Press* [26]

"The state has fined a hospital $11,000 in the death of a 10-month-old boy who authorities say was given an overdose of medication because his doctor had omitted a decimal point in his instructions."
– *Associated Press* [27]

See if you can find the contradiction in the next two articles found one month apart:

"The National Institute of Health showed estrogen not only improves cholesterol levels, but also reduces the risk of blood clots that can cause heart attacks." – *CNN* [28]

"Use of estrogen treatment may increase a woman's chance of developing breast cancer." – *CNN* [29]

It's your choice ... would you prefer heart disease or breast cancer?

A few years later it seems they have changed their mind:

"Hormone-replacement therapy, widely believed to be an effective treatment for heart ailments in older women, does not appreciably slow progression of cardiac disease, researchers at Wake Forest University have found." – *CNN* [30]

Or how about the incongruity in these two articles:

"The risk of kidney failure appeared to be doubled by either heavy average use (more than 365 pills per year) or moderate cumulative use (more than 1000 pills in a lifetime.)" – *Associated Press* [31]

"Taking an aspirin every other day for 20 years can cut your risk of colon cancer nearly in half, a study suggests." (Note: Over 3,650 aspirins in a lifetime!) – *Associated Press* [32]

By following the advice of one researcher to reduce your risk of colon cancer you subject yourself to the dangerous effects of kidney and liver disease. These contradictions are epidemic in the field of medicine and pharmacology.

One of the most dramatic and heart-wrenching stories I have seen was in the *Boston Globe* in March 1995:

"When an award-winning health columnist for one of the biggest newspapers in the country got breast cancer, she went to one of the best hospitals in the world. The *Boston Globe's* Betsy Lehman, of all people, wound up dead because of a huge mistake at the Dana-Farber Cancer Institute, of all places. The fatal mistake, disclosed Thursday by the *Globe* was the latest in a series of blatant medical errors that have hurt the reputation of some of America's best hospitals and alarmed patients. Lehman's heart failed after she was given four times the maximum safe dosage of a highly toxic drug during chemotherapy. At least a dozen doctors, nurses, and pharmacists overlooked the error for four days while Lehman continued to receive an overdose of cyclophosphamide, and a four-fold overdose of another drug meant to shield her from side effects. 'She was dealing with horrendous symptoms,' Lehman's husband, Robert Distel, a scientist at Dana Farber, told the *Globe*, 'The whole lining of her gut from one end to the other was shedding. She was vomiting sheets of tissue. They said that this was the worse they'd ever seen. But the doctors said it was normal.' Lehman, a 39-year-old mother of two, died Dec. 3. An Autopsy found no visible signs of cancer in her body. The mistake wasn't discovered until February 13, after clerks went through records."[33]

When you read stories like this you begin to wonder what we can trust in regards to our health-care. In my files, I have literally thousands of such articles. And in my life I too, have a similar story.

When I was about five-years-old, my older brother Marc broke his arm. My father rushed him to the hospital and I went along for the ride. After my brother was x-rayed, we were brought into an examination/treatment room where we waited ... and waited ... and waited. Finally, a doctor arrived and examined my brother's arm. He then proceeded to wrap his arm in a bandage coated with plaster of paris which was to be a cast. My father was discussing my brother's condition and the necessary home-care procedures with the doctor when my brother interrupted, "Dad?"

My father replied, "Not now, Marc," and continued his conversation.

After a few more moments, my brother again interrupted, "Dad!?"

"Not Now Marc!" my father again replied, this time with a tone of anger in his voice. He continued his discussion with the doctor.

Finally, my brother yelled, "DAD!!!"

"WHAT?!" my father yelled back.

My brother explained his interruptions with frustration, "The doctor is putting the cast on the wrong arm."

This example may not be as extreme as many that occur, however, it seems the one thing we can truly trust in our healing process is the innate healer within ourselves. Within our bodies lies the world's largest drugstore. Our bodies contain an immense healing potential which if we align ourselves with it and pay heed to its signals, health and well-being are certain.

A Note on Antibiotics

One of the most misunderstood and overused medical treatments available to the health-care consumer today is antibiotics. When an individual begins to experience symptoms such as fever, diarrhea, nausea and aches, it is very common to run to their family doctor and get a prescription for antibiotics. What is unfortunate is, that many doctors prescribe these drugs merely as a procedure of protocol whether they will benefit the patient or not, often to merely console the patient.

According to an article in the *Palm Beach Post* in September of 1997, "...doctors wrote 12 million antibiotic prescriptions in a single year for colds, bronchitis and other respiratory infection against which the drugs are almost always useless.

"Such indiscriminate use of antibiotics has contributed to the emergence of drug resistant bacteria, a growing problem in the United States. More than 90 percent of upper respiratory infections, including bronchitis and colds are caused by a virus and are therefore impervious to antibiotics. Doctors usually know this, but studies have suggested they may yield to pressure from patients – or what they perceive to be the patients' expectations – to prescribe a drug, even if it is unlikely to help."[34]

The word *Antibiotic* means "to destroy life."[35] They are not selective in what life they destroy. When you take an antibiotic, it goes to work to destroy anything living, whether it is a bacteria or a human cell. Antibiotics are very dangerous and often have no beneficial effect on the body.

According to recent studies, the typical flu, left on its own, generally resolves itself within three to five days, whereas if you take antibiotics it can last 10 to 14 days.[36]

Why is this? All symptoms of the flu are created by the body in order to heal. If these processes are allowed to express themselves fully, the flu is eliminated. Medications such as antibiotics, aspirin and other symptom relievers interfere with these processes prolonging the flu. So why are antibiotics prescribed? Because that is what the medical protocol dictates, teaches, and ultimately, what patients demand. Dr. Ralph Gonzales of the University of Colorado Health Sciences Center has great advice, "Give your body's own immune system enough time to clear the infection."[37]

In outlining the fifth cause of our health-care crisis I hope I have revealed to you the fallacy of the scientific method, for in their search for strict objective data, they have lost sight of that which does the healing ... the human spirit. In the chapters that follow, you will discover that the moments of greatest healing are unexplained by medical science and labeled as "spontaneous remission," "medical miracles," and "unexplained phenomenon." The truth is that healing will never result from objective, clinical, scientific trials. Healing is a subjective, self-created experience. In the words of Dr. Donald Epstein, "Healing is an inside job."[38]

CAUSE #6

Separation and Segregation

When we look at the world around us, it appears that it is composed of individual parts. When we look at ourselves, it seems to our senses that we are all separate and different. This experience and perception of *separation* is a false precept in spite of its seemingly obvious reality. "Of course, I am separate from everything else in the world," you might say, "I am here, that is there and you are over there." This world-view is easily accepted, for on the surface it appears to be this way to our five senses, yet when we learn the truth, we see that all things are manifestations of one united universe. In fact, the word Uni-verse means "one turn" or "one song."[39]

This divided mentality has extended into every aspect of our lives and society. Most affected by this false notion is our health-care system. When we view the body as a collection of parts, it is inevitable that more disease will ensue. Disease is the experience of separateness within. When our organs and cells work independently of one another, we experience disease. The best example of this is cancer.

Cancer is the experience of a collection of human cells functioning independently of the rest of the body. It is a renegade band of human tissue acting on their own accord, regardless of its effect on the rest of the body. Only when we create unity and harmony within the cells and organs of the body can the diseased part become one with the rest of the body. Only then will the body become whole or, in other words, heal.

It is this "separation" manner of thinking that leads to its dark predecessor, "segregation." *Segregation* is the mechanism by which anger, fear or hatred is expressed and acted upon an apparent *other*. It is the view that this "other" is different than myself, wrong, and therefore a threat. This "threat" must be separated from us even further and, if at all possible, destroyed. It is this process by which all prejudice, crime, war and racial cleansing is based. This mentality only leads to destruction and further separation and disease.

The sad thing about this is that the two institutions that are responsible for the welfare of our nation's community – the Health-Care industry and the Criminal Rehabilitation establishment – both function on the level of separation and segregation. In these institutions, the thought process is as follows, "Let's find the bad, diseased individual that is disturbing the rest of the community and control, remove or destroy them."

It may appear that removing a sick individual from the collective is a viable solution, but it is a futile effort. The reason this individual has become diseased is that it was separate to begin with. This sick part acts defiantly in an effort to become one with the collective. As long as we continue to view our ailments (whether within ourselves or outside in our community) from a segregated and separated mentality, we will continue to have disease in our bodies and crime in our streets.

If instead, we welcome that diseased part back into our collective selves, and realize that only through re-establishing harmonious relationships among individuals, can we begin to experience wholeness, healing and health.

As Neale Donald Walsch so eloquently stated, "There is only one of us in the room."[40] It is only through this understanding that we will bring greater healing to us as individuals and to the world.

CAUSE #7

Disempowering Belief Systems

The seventh and most important cause of our health-care crisis is our tendency to hold onto old *belief systems* based on outdated science and cultural superstition. I have found that there are seven beliefs inhibiting healing and growth, keeping us in the situation that we now find ourselves – spending more money with more people getting sick.

We have begun to understand the cause of our current health-care crisis. Now, we can dig deeper and uncover these inner beliefs, both individually and collectively, that are the basis of these seven causes. In the next chapter, we will investigate in depth the seven belief systems that inhibit healing and have contributed to our current health-care crisis. Through this awareness we can begin to let go of these disempowering and unserving beliefs and establish new, empowering beliefs. After each one of these beliefs have been examined, I have suggested alternative beliefs based on current scientific knowledge and ancient spiritual wisdom, that are used to stimulate healing and support the expression of our optimum potential. In chapter 5, A New Vision of Truth, the universal principles and laws upon which these new beliefs are based will be elaborated and demonstrated to transform these beliefs into something much greater ... knowing.

1. Langford, Jerome J., Galileo, *Science and The Church*, Ann Arbor, MI, University of Michigan Press, 1996, p.55.
2. Langford, ibid, pp. 152-154
3. Morison, Samuel Eliot, *Christopher Columbus*, Mariner, Meridian Books, 1992.
4. "True adventure harder to find," *USA Today*, October 19, 1999.
5. Dubos, René, *Pasteur and Modern Science*, Doubleday and Co.,Inc., New York, 1960
6. James, Walene, *Immunization: The Reality Behind the Myth*, Bergin & Garvey, New York, 1988, pp. 23-38
7. Miller, Neil Z., *Vaccines: Are They Really Safe and Effective*, New Atlantean Press, Figure 1
8. Friend, Tim, "Vaccine caused almost all polio since '80," *USA Today*
9. Miller, ibid., Figures 5 & 7.

10. Cournoyer, Cynthia, *What About Immunization? Exposing The Vaccine Philosophy*, Dennis Nelson Publishing, pp. 36-43.
11. Cournoyer, ibid.
12. Clark, Amy Rosenbaum, "A Dilemma Over DTP," *Vegetarian Times*, September 1994, p.98.
13. Cournoyer, ibid.
14. Fisher, Barbara Loe, "Shots in the Dark," *The Next City*, Volume 4, Number 4, Summer 1999, pp. 33-39, 45-47, 52-55.
15. Wallechinsky, David, et.al., *Book of Lists*, William Morrow and Company, New York, 1977, p. 469.
16. "Drugs and Other Medical Nondurables Expenditures and Average Annual Percent Change, by *Source of Funds*: Selected Calendar Years 1970-2008," Health Care Financing Administration, Office of the Actuary., http://www.hcfa.gov/stats/NHE-Proj/proj1998/tables/table11a.htm
17. Pastore, Michael, "Non-Violently Give Up Your Television," *Brief New World*, http://www.cpsweb.com/youthtopia/1b022299.htm
18. Pert, Candice, Ph.D., *Molecules of Emotion*, Simon & Schuster, 1999.
19. Pearce, Joseph Chilton, *The Crack in the Cosmic Egg*, Julian Press, New York, 1973, pp. 63-70.
20. "Where is the wisdom...? The poverty of medical evidence," *British Medical Journal*, Volume 303, October 5, 1991, p.798.
21. Leape, Lucian L., M.D., "Error in Medicine," *Journal of the American Medical Association*, Volume 272, No. 23, December 21, 1994, p. 1851.
22. Starfield, Barbara, MD, MPH, "Is US Health Really the Best in the World," *Journal of the American Medical Institution*, Volume 284, Number 4, July 26, 2000.
23. ibid.
24. Saal JS, et al. "Nonoperative management of herniated cervical intervertebral disc with radiculopathy." *Spine*. 1996 Aug 15;21(16):1877-83.
25. Friend, Tim, "Human error clouds results of mammograms," *USA Today*, December 1, 1994
26. Griffen, Laura, "Fort Worth hospital settles lung suit," *Dallas Morning News*, April 2, 1995, p. 38A.
27. "Hospital fined in fatal overdose," *Boston Globe*, October 7, 1998.
28. "Study reinforces that estrogen may reduce heart risks," *CNN*, Washington, March 5, 1997.
29. "New study links estrogen treatment and breast cancer," *CNN*, Washington, February 26, 1997.
30. "Hormone therapy fails to slow heart disease in older women, study finds," *CNN*, Los Angeles, March 13, 2000.
31. "Pain Pill Research: Overuse linked to kidney damage," *Newsweek*, December 22, 1994, pp A7, A57.
32. Giovannucci E, Rimm E, et al. "Aspirin Use and the Risk for Colorectal Cancer and Adenoma in Male Health Professionals." *Annals of Internal Medicine* 1994 Aug. 15; pp 241-46.
33. "Hospital error fatal for notable columnist," *The Express Times*, March 24, 1995.
34. "12 Million Rx's for antibiotics useless", *Palm Beach Post*, September 17, 1997, p. 12A.
35. *Webster's Seventh New Collegiate Dictionary*, G.&C. Merrium Co., 1965, p. 38.
36. Friend, Tim, "Parents give kids useless risky drugs," *USA Today*, October 5, 1994.
37. See [33], ibid.
38. Epstein, Donald, *The 12 Stages of Healing: A Network Approach to Wellness*, Amber-Allen Publishing, 1994.
39. *Webster's Seventh New Collegiate Dictionary*, G.&C. Merrium Co., 1965, p. 971.
40. Walsch, Neale Donald, *Conversations with God*, Hampton Roads Publishing, 1995.

Exposing The Crisis : Summary

The United States is currently in a health-care crisis in which we are spending more money each year on health-care, yet the population in general is becoming sicker. There are seven causes to this health-care crisis:

1. **Lack of Responsibility** – The general public is uneducated in making appropriate decisions and in taking charge of their own health.
2. **Encouraged Apathy** – There is a pattern of not caring within the general public which is encouraged by the corporate world of health-care.
3. **Unwavering Traditionalism** – People tend to hold on to traditional ideas resisting change and new paradigms of belief.
4. **Nurtured Fear** – The corporate world also sponsors fear as a motivating force to keep the general public in their market share.
5. **Objective Dogma** – The belief that all things real must be measurable.
6. **Segregation and Separation** – Disease is a result of separation within our bodies. Often the treatment of this disease, both individually and socially, creates further separation known as segregation. Healing is the process of becoming whole.
7. **Disempowering Belief Systems** – There are a number of belief systems which encourage dis-ease and inhibit healing.

4

LIFTING THE VEIL OF ILLUSION

Maintaining order rather than correcting disorder
Is the ultimate principle of wisdom.
To cure disease after it has appeared,
Is like digging a well when one already feels thirsty,
Or forging a weapon after the war has already begun.
~ Nei Jing
2nd Century Chinese Medical Classic

Throughout my years in practice, and speaking with thousands of people, I have found that there are seven core beliefs, or what I like to call *illusions*, that inhibit healing and actually promote disease. These illusions are outdated and old-fashioned beliefs created by old science and ancient superstition. They promote fear amongst their believers, and disempower them from living to their fullest potential. However, once these illusions are exposed and acknowledged, the individual realizes the naiveté and ignorance of this failing notion, and immediately experiences a sense of expansion and relief. With the understanding of true principle, healing spontaneously results.

This chapter offers an alternative belief to each of the seven illusions. The following chapter explains in more depth, the principles upon which these new beliefs are founded. But first, let's look at the illusions of our current health-care system.

ILLUSION #1

The Illusion of the Victim

> *"Disease and health come from outside of me.*
> *I am merely a victim of circumstance."*

We believe that illness and disease come from outside of ourselves, from a hostile environment in the form of bacteria, viruses, germs, toxins, allergens, and stress.

As demonstrated earlier, if there is a pile of cow manure in a field with flies swarming around it, are the flies the problem, or is it the mess in the field? You can swat the flies all you want, but if you don't clean up the mess, nothing you do, will get rid of the flies. The flies are innocent.

So are the germs in your body. They are opportunists that take advantage of any poor soul who allows garbage to collect in their bodies or minds. Even Pasteur, the developer of the Germ Theory said on his deathbed, "It's not the germ, it's the soil."

Germs, bacteria, viruses, toxins, as well as stress, are not the cause of disease. Our body's inability to cope with them is. Therefore, disease does not come from out there, but from within ourselves ... and so does health.

New Belief: "I am the cause of everything in my life."

ILLUSION #2

The Illusion of Possession

> *"I have an illness."*

It is a common belief that when we are ill, we *have* a disease. This belief has been promoted and suggested through the allopathic model of diagnosis and treatment. Because of this model, the American public and much of the world, has come to a false understanding that diseases are something we catch, we have, and we must dispossess ourselves of. Physical ailments such as cancer, diabetes and arthritis, as examples, are contracted and caught, at which time we then have that disease. The disease then must be identified, labeled with a diagnosis, at which time it can be treated, and hopefully cured. More severe developmental and behavioral conditions, such as autism, cerebral palsy and multiple sclerosis, are also conditions that we *have.* This concept of having a condition, disease or ailment, runs the gamut of medical diagnoses ... and is an illusion. These diagnoses serve only to continue apathy and fear in our society, and the treatment of these conditions seldom results in health or healing.

All disease is created from within, in response to changes in the environment known as stresses, or due to the inability to adapt appropriately to stress. Healing takes place through the recovery of this adaptation, or through the restoration of the ability to respond. The inside-out approach to identifying illness is an illusion, so too, is the outside-in treatment of disease a futile effort.

In truth, there is no disease known to man, that isn't created, developed and maintained in existence by the body and mind of the individual who is experiencing it. Every disease that is presently documented in medical texts, as well as those not yet discovered are adaptive responses to changes in the environment. It is a moment of healing, so as to prevent death and sustain life.

New Belief: "I am experiencing a healing process."

ILLUSION #3

The Illusion of Permanence

"Same 'ol same 'ol. Nothing ever changes."

When we look at our bodies, a table, or any other physical object, it appears solid and immobile. When we have an injured part or sick organ, we feel helpless. We feel we are stuck with it forever and that we will suffer till our last dying day.

This is an illusion. Our bodies are ever-changing. The cells of our body are constantly being sloughed off and replaced with new ones every day. All the atoms, elements and molecules, that make up our cells are in a constant exchange with the outside environment.

According to Dr. Deepak Chopra, in his book, *Perfect Health*, "The Greek philosopher Heraclitus declared, 'You cannot step into the same river twice, for fresh waters are ever flowing in.' The same is true of the body. If you 'pinch an inch' around your waist, the fat you are squeezing between your fingers is not the same as it was last month. The adipose tissues (fat cells) fill up with fat and empty out constantly, so that all of it is exchanged every three weeks. You acquire a new stomach lining every five days (the innermost layer of stomach cells is exchanged in a matter of minutes as you digest food). Your skin renews itself every five weeks. Your skeleton, seemingly so solid and rigid, is entirely new every three months. In all, the flow of oxygen, carbon, hydrogen, and nitrogen is so rapid that you could be renewed in a matter of weeks ... "

He goes on to say, "You appear to be the same outwardly, yet you are like a building whose bricks are constantly being replaced by new ones. Every year, 98 percent of the total number of atoms in your body are replaced ... confirmed by radioisotope studies at the Oak Ridge laboratories in California."[1]

Your body is not as solid and unchanging as you thought. With the right actions, no matter your condition or illness, you can have a brand new body by the same time next year.

New Belief: "My life and body are in a constant state of change, transformation and evolution."

ILLUSION #4

The Illusion of Helplessness

"There is nothing I can do."

When we are in a state of crisis or illness, we feel helpless. We feel as if there is nothing we can do. It is common for a suffering individual to come to my office with tears in their eyes or anger in their hearts and plead with me to just make it go away.

Whenever something unfavorable happens in our life, such as a physical illness, loss of a job, or break-up in a relationship, we feel that it was our fault and that we did something wrong. We blame ourselves and our self-esteem withers away. We lose confidence in ourselves, and cast our inner strength and power into the sea of despair. In this state of mind, we don't have the power to change and we dwindle into helplessness.

In regards to health-care, it has been driven into our brains that when we are sick, we go to the doctor. We are told over and over again, through drug advertisements on television, that if we are feeling under the weather or experience any sign of sickness in the form of symptoms, we can travel to our local pharmacy or supermarket and visit the over-the-counter drug aisle for our relief. Likewise, if we are feeling anxious ... the psychotherapist; our back hurts ... the chiropractor; our child has a fever ... the pediatrician. The list goes on and on.

What I want you to understand is not that these professionals are bad – they aren't. In fact, I think they are wonderful and valuable members of our society. The only danger in utilizing their services, is when we *freely* hand over our inner power to them and say, "Fix me." Healing can only occur when we experience a greater wholeness within and become aware of our healing power.

By placing our lives in their hands, blindly accepting what they wish to say or do to us, we enter into a codependent relationship with them – a relationship in which two parties become dependent on each other's existence and cannot survive without the other.[2]

In the case of the professional and the client, the client depends solely on the professional to save them when they are in trouble, and the professional depends on the client to pay them. This is not a bad thing if the person is seriously in crisis; however, when the crisis has abated the client must regain control of his or her life. This is often not the case, and the client continues to rely on the professional as their savior.

There is a better, healthier way. When we understand that all healing comes from within, and we each have the power to grow, evolve and become better, we look at our healing professionals in a different light. Rather than looking at them as our saving grace, we see them as teachers and healing facilitators from whom we seek council. By using their services to provide information, we can accept responsibility and take the appropriate actions. The word doctor literally means "teacher," and the word professional is defined as "one who professes, or declares wisdom or knowledge."[3] I believe the holders of these titles, as well as those who seek their services, have forgotten this. The only person anyone can heal ... is themselves.

New Belief: "I have the power and ability to heal myself."

ILLUSION #5

The Illusion of Scarcity and Failure

"My body makes mistakes that need to be fixed."

Do any of these statements sound familiar: "My bad back," "My stomach problem," "My malignant...," "My head is killing me." How about these: "I need an aspirin." "Where's my blood pressure medication?" "I have to go in for surgery."

All of these statements are based on the illusion that our body doesn't have a clue as to what it's doing and must constantly be fixed.

This is an illusion. Our bodies are infinitely intelligent. Each one of us has vast wisdom. Right now, as you read these words your heart is pumping, sending blood and oxygen to all parts of your body; your stomach and digestive system are digesting your last meal, breaking apart the food into its molecular components and distributing them to the proper channels; your liver and kidneys are filtering your blood and other fluids, removing all the toxins from your body; your immune system is keeping your body clear of dangerous bacteria, viruses, and other opportunistic varmints; and over a million organized, on-purpose chemical reactions are occurring every second.

How can your body do all that, every moment and yet you can still concentrate on what you are reading? The answer is your body is so intelligent that it does all this without any conscious thought on your part. Not to say *you* are separate from your body and its activity. This is all you, being you.

Everything your body does is with the purpose of keeping you alive, healthy, and moving towards greater health and ability.

What about symptoms? What about headaches, back pain, fever, swelling, itching, vomiting, diarrhea, and fatigue? These are all intelligent body functions maintaining our health. Pain alerts us to problems in the body. Fever is our body's way of destroying bacteria, viruses, and toxins – it cooks them. Swelling brings the immune system's white blood cells to an infected or injured area. Itching is the sensation of old cells being replaced by the new. Diarrhea and vomiting are the body's method of removing *dangerous stuff* from our bodies that might otherwise kill us. Fatigue is our body telling us to rest. Everything that our body does is for a reason.

The next time you experience a symptom or illness, rather than saying, "Why me? Make it go away," ask yourself, "What is my body trying to accomplish and what can I do to support the process?"

New Belief: *"My body has an innate intelligence that does not need help, only freedom from interference."*

ILLUSION #6

The Illusion of Separation

"I am separate from the world and others."

When we look at ourselves and the world around us, it appears that we are separate from everything that surrounds us. We look in the mirror and say, "This is my body – my arms, my legs. I am a separate individual." On the surface, this observation would appear correct.

This is an illusion. All things in the universe are interconnected as one whole. In the new avenues of physics and quantum mechanics, it has been confirmed that within the deepest levels of ourselves and the world around us, there is an infinite world of energy and vibration that unites all things into one cohesive whole.

To get a clearer picture answer the question: Where does the air in your bedroom end and the air in your living room begin? or, the air inside your house and the air outside? or the air in your lungs and the air outside your body? or the air in Davenport, Iowa and the air in Chang Mai, Thailand? There is no separation.

Like the air, our bodies, and all other physical objects, are just different vibrations and *clumps* of the energy that pervades all of existence. We have the *Universe* ... the uni-verse ... literally, one turn ... one vibration ... one word ... one song.

New Belief: *"The Universe and I are one."*

ILLUSION #7

The Illusion of The Cure

"Something or someone out there will heal me."

Thanks to the never-ending bombardment of television drug commercials and the medical dogma of "the cure," many people believe that the answer to their health-concerns is out there somewhere in the form of a pill, lotion, potion, treatment, therapy, or surgery. This is an illusion.

Healing is an inside job. If you put a bandage over a cut on your finger, does the bandage do the healing? Absolutely not. It absorbs any blood and prevents the injury from becoming dirty, while the body heals the wound. The body sends white blood cells to the area to fight any infectious invaders. The blood clots, and the wound begins to close as a scab, and before you know it the skin is replaced, the finger prints intact.

This is the miraculous healing potential of the body at work. Yet, it does not stop with a simple wound. It is this innate healer within each of us that mends the broken bone (while the cast merely holds the bone in position), rids our body of the common cold or influenza, and heals us of diseases such as cancer and hypertension.

Most importantly, when we visit a doctor, therapist, or any of the many alternative health practitioners, we often surrender ourselves to their "healing" hands with the hope and faith that they will heal us. While it is important to surrender to the service they provide, there is a major distinction that must be made: The only person an individual can heal is themselves.

If these individuals tell you that they will cure or heal you, they are either deceiving you or are unaware of true healing. They are, in truth, healing facilitators. They are supporting you in your healing process.

Remember these words: *You are the Healer!* A true doctor or healing facilitator will always empower you and remind you of this fact. Beware of those who claim to be your healer. Their services will only work to disempower you. They, like you, can only heal themselves, and in cases such as these, the only thing they will heal is their ego.

New Belief: "All healing comes from within."

This chapter has explained to you, what I believe are the seven beliefs that inhibit healing and that have created what we now call the health-care crisis. I have also offered seven new beliefs, that will inspire and promote healing, and will create a solution that will result in a true health-care system, rather than the disease-care system we currently are employing.

Let's continue our journey and explore current scientific knowledge, derived from such fields of study such as quantum physics, relativity theory, and psychology. This exploration will give us a solid foundation of understanding, making these new beliefs believable.

1.   Chopra, Deepak, *Perfect Health*, Harmony Books, 1991, p. 12.
2.   Bradshaw, John, *Homecoming*, Bantam, 1990, pp 8-9.
3.   *Webster's Seventh New Collegiate Dictionary*, G.&C. Merrium Co., 1965, p. 245, 680.

Lifting the Veil of Illusion: Summary

There are seven core beliefs, or illusions, inherent in our culture that inhibit healing and encourage dis-ease. Here are seven new beliefs to inspire and encourage healing.

1. **The Illusion of the Victim** – "Disease and Health come from outside me. I am a victim of circumstance."
   New Belief: I am the cause of everything in my life.

2. **The Illusion of Possession** – "I have an illness."
   New Belief: I am experiencing a healing process

3. **The Illusion of Permanence** – "Same ol' Same ol.' Nothing ever changes."
   New Belief: My life and body are in a constant state of change, transformation, and evolution.

4. **The Illusion of Helplessness** – "There is nothing I can do."
   New Belief: I have the power and ability to heal myself.

5. **The Illusion of Scarcity and Failure** – "My body makes mistakes which need to be fixed."
   New Belief: My body has an innate intelligence which needs no help ... just no interference.

6. **The Illusion of Separation** – "I am separate from the world and others."
   New Belief: The Universe and I are one.

7. **The Illusion of the Cure** – "Something or someone out there will heal me."
   New Belief: All healing comes from within.

PART II

OFF THE BEATEN PATH

5

A NEW VISION OF TRUTH
The Seven Universal Healing Principles

*You cannot solve a problem, with the same level
of consciousness that created it.* ~ *Albert Einstein*

*A mind stretched by a new idea never returns
to its original dimensions.* ~ *Oliver Wendell Holmes*

In our quest for health and healing we have revealed and acknowledged the things inhibiting healing. We examined the causes of our current health-care crisis, as well as the belief systems, or illusions, that prevent healing from occurring, and learned new beliefs that are supportive of health.

Now we will explore the seven principles upon which these new beliefs are founded. These principles were originally revealed through the intuitive wisdom of ancient sages and spiritual teachers and have been passed down to those seeking to benefit from their gifts. Our modern-day sages, the physicists, with the advent of quantum mechanics and relativity, have affirmed these notions and now accept them as fact.

These principles govern everything in the universe. They are the natural laws of which all things must and do follow. These laws dictate how things come into existence, as well as how they behave once arisen. These truths maintain all things in reality and determine when they cease to be. If you learn these principles, believe these truths, and follow these laws, all things that you desire, including optimum, vibrant health, will be yours. The more we think and act in opposition of these seven principles, the further we will find ourselves from our hopes; however, if we put ourselves in alignment with these truths, the more our lives will reflect our greatest dreams.

HEALING PRINCIPLE #1

The Law of Cause and Effect

All things in existence have a cause. Everything in the universe was caused by something else. Whether it is a wave in the ocean, a wind between the leaves of an oak or the thought in a little boy's mind, all things are the effects of another cause. Every cause has an effect, and every effect will be the cause of something else. An apple, for example, is the effect of a fruiting tree. The tree is the effect of a germinated seed, whose cause was another apple. The cycle of cause and effect is infinite and eternal and is the fundamental principle upon which everything in the universe functions ... including healing.

Throughout the ages, our great spiritual and philosophical masters have taught us that if there is a certain effect you desire, there are certain causes that must be initiated to manifest that desire. If you wish an apple tree, you must plant a seed. If you wish to win the love of another, you must express your love to them. If you wish to create something new, you must first create the idea in your mind. All things have a cause. If you know what you wish to create, and you know its cause, all you must do is put that cause into action and the effect of your desire is guaranteed ... including optimum health and well-being.

No matter what it is you wish to manifest in your life, there are three basic causes in this universe – *thoughts*, *words* and *actions*. Everything in existence was at one time an idea. Look at the book you are reading. Look at the chair in which you sit. Look at the hand that holds the book. All of these things were at one time an idea in someone's mind. This book had to be conceived, then typed, and finally, printed on paper. The chair needed to be designed and crafted in wood. Your hand is the result of the loving union of a man and woman who, together, decided to have a child. All things in the universe were once a thought, brought into reality through vibration and motion ... word and action.

If all things have a cause, then what is the cause of thought? What is the cause of an idea? The cause of all thoughts and ideas is *intention*. It is through intention that we think about what we wish to create. Through this thought we might express our ideas into written words and take the appropriate actions.

The cause of intention is Desire. What is the cause of desire? As Wallace Wattles says in the 1902 classic, *The Science of Getting Rich*, "All desire is either possibility seeking expression or function seeking performance."[1]

We may then ask, "What is the cause of possibility and function?" The search for ultimate cause has intrigued the human mind throughout our existence and drives all spiritual practice and scientific investigation. I prefer to believe that there is an ultimate intelligence from which all possibility, function, desire and intention arise, and it is from this intention that all things in the universe manifest. You might call this God. You might call this the Unified Field of energy and matter. You may call it Universal Intelligence, Hunab Ku, Tao, Brahma, or Allah. It doesn't matter what you call it, or if you call it at all, there must be a primary cause (unless, of course, there isn't.)

Although the expression of thought through words and actions does speed up the manifestation process, all that is needed to express possibility or perform function is desire and intention. It is through intention and desire that everything is created and made to manifest.

In the current health-care model of which we find ourselves today, there is a backwards philosophy of treatment where the effects are attacked through chemical or surgical means. If there is a headache or fever, take an aspirin to make it go away. If we have nausea or diarrhea, take that pink stuff to make it go away. If we have allergies or a cough, take allergy or cough medicine – you guessed it – to make it go away. Do we ever ask the questions: Why are we experiencing these symptoms? or, What is the cause?

The problem with this model is that they are attempting to create a different effect altering a false cause. As discussed earlier, bacteria and viruses are not the cause of disease. They are the effect of a weakened, susceptible environment, collectively; our body, thoughts, words and actions or intentions.

Is the headache caused by a deficiency of aspirin, or the nausea caused by an absence of pink stuff? I think not. By changing the misrepresented cause, the effect will not change. Until your beliefs, thoughts and intentions are in alignment with the natural laws and the principles of health, nothing you can say or do will bring that which you desire ... health, happiness, prosperity and the fullest expression of who you are.

This principle, or *law of cause and effect* is unwavering in its expression. Remember, for every effect a cause ... and every cause an effect. The cause will always produce its effect and the effect will always be produced by its cause.

By taking medication with the sole purpose to make the symptom, or effect, go away is like blowing at the smoke to put out the fire. We are numbing the signal for change without acknowledging its purpose or cause. Every symptom has a purpose. As stated earlier, fever destroys bacteria, viruses and toxins, nausea and vomiting remove dangerous substances from our bodies and pain alerts us to potential danger. If we were to maintain our automobile with this same mentality we would find ourselves quickly stuck on the side of the road.

In a vitalistic model of health-care, we ask a different question. What is my body trying to accomplish by manifesting this symptom and what can I do to support it?

We must accept responsibility and take the appropriate actions to cause our desired effect – health and healing. Health and disease do not come by accident. They are definite effects of definite causes.

If we decide on the effects we desire in our lives, we can study and acquire the knowledge of what causes those effects, and take the appropriate actions based on this knowledge, then health is inevitable.

This is the first principle of healing. Every effect has a cause ... and that cause always produces that effect. No exceptions. If there is a condition, situation or person in your life that is disagreeable or not exactly to your liking, some thought, word or action was expressed in the past to bring about this effect. By acknowledging and accepting this fact, you now have the power to perceive (the first attribute of health) the cause that produced this effect, and then at that moment, begin to create a new thought, word and/or action to create a new experience in the future. As the great motivational speaker Anthony Robbins advocated, "The past does not equal the future."[2]

If we want to create health and healing (the effects) in our lives, we first must learn the causes. If we are to experience vibrant, abundant health in our lives, we must learn what thoughts, words, and actions we must take in order to create it in our lives. In chapter 6, you'll learn the seven attributes of health. In chapter 8, you'll learn the seven powers of the mind and how to use thought and speech to create health, or that which you desire. In chapter 9, you will explore the role of emotions in healing and how they effect our health and healing process. And in chapter 11, you will learn the seven responsibilities, or actions, which if implemented will insure a lifetime of vibrant health and enjoyment.

HEALING PRINCIPLE #2

The Law of Energy and Vibration

It has been proven that all things in the universe are composed of pure energy. The physical world that we see, hear and feel are all manifestations of energy. Look at your hand. It looks solid enough. Examine the lines and contours created by the skin prints, veins and bones. Study the colors and tones of the skin and the blood vessels beneath. When we look at the skin, it appears as one expansive, continuous sheet that covers our entire body without break or separation.

Yet, when you look at the skin under a microscope, you find that it is not one sheet at all. It is composed of millions of individual components called cells, all working together to create this living thing called skin. Every organ and part of the body including the heart, brain, liver and bone, are likewise composed of these individual cells.

Each one of these cells is a complex organism in and of itself. When we look at a human skin cell it is a world within a world. Within each cell, are organelles or sub-cells that have separate functions such as waste disposal, energy production and the most magnificent component of all, genetic potential. These cells and their sub-cellular components, look like solid structures, yet when we examine them closer we find that they are made up of even smaller components called molecules.

Molecules are chemical substances that give the physical world its properties and functions. Yet these structures, when examined closer, are also made up of even smaller structures called atoms – the basic building block of physical matter.

These atoms are also composed of smaller subatomic components. The atom is like a tiny microscopic solar system similar to our sun and its planets. In the center is a sun-like nucleus of protons and neutrons around which planet-like electrons orbit at blinding speeds nearing the speed of light. Between this central nucleus and its orbiting electrons lies empty space, so vast, that relative to the size of these tiny particles, the space is greater than the size of our entire solar system.

When we examine these subatomic particles, we discover something truly amazing – they are not composed of even smaller components – they are concentrated clouds of pure energy. Everything that appears solid and dense are in their essential state, constructed from concentrated clouds of energy spinning at blinding speeds in vast expanses of empty space.

With this perspective and understanding, look at your hand. No longer do we need to be trapped by the illusion of solidity, but instead, we are mesmerized by the notion that we are examining energy and space.

By doing this exercise, we learn to appreciate the true nature of our physical world. All things in existence in our universe are made up of energy. Make a fist and knock on something solid such as a wooden desk or a metal door. It seems solid and stable, yet, in truth, it is pure energy and space.

Now, this energy is not still. It is in constant movement. In fact, everything in the universe is constantly moving. We call this movement vibration. Atoms and subatomic energy particles are in a constant, eternal vibrational motion. Whether they are moving back and forth like a pendulum or spinning like a top, the concentrated energy that makes up all things is constantly moving. When we look at the wooden desk or the metal door, we have a new perception as to their true nature. They are composed of energy that is constantly moving through vast areas of space. It is our perception that creates the reality of solidity which is interpreted from the signals sent to our brain by our senses – an illusion concocted by our inner filters. Its true nature is energy and vibration.

Our five senses are vibrational receivers. Our eyes, ears, nose, tongue and touch senses are antennas that are calibrated to different frequencies, or speeds of vibration. Our brain and nervous system are vibration-interpreting and reality-creating computers. Our experiences are the interpretive expression of a never-ending cascade of vibration. Let's look at a few examples.

If I look at an apple, what I am seeing is my own interpretation of vibration. Light waves that reflect off the mass of energy we have collectively called an apple enters my eye through the dark round opening called the pupil. The light vibration energy impacts light-sensitive cells called rods and cones, in the back of my eye. These cells are reactive to light converting the vibration into an electrical signal. The electrical signal travels along the optic nerve to the brain where it is translated into an image, and we experience sight – specifically, what we have come to know as an apple.

Likewise, when listening to a symphony or hearing a noise, these sounds are vibrations traveling through the air. When these vibrations strike my ear drum, it too vibrates. These vibrations are then transferred to tiny hairs within the inner ear that stimulate the acoustic nerve. The nerve again converts this into an electrical signal that is carried to the brain where it is translated into our experience of hearing.

By understanding this, we view our world in a new and liberating way.

How can we apply this knowledge to aid our quest for health and healing? When we understand that our seemingly permanent injury, illness or condition is an expression of *energy and vibration*, it creates a sense of impermanence and change. That is the basis of the next Principle of Healing.

HEALING PRINCIPLE #3

The Law of Perpetual Change

Everything in the universe is in a constant state of change. Nothing remains the same. Whether we are discussing a solid piece of stone, a sheet of steel, a mighty oak or the thoughts in our heads, everything is changing. *The only thing constant, is change.*

Our universe and all of its constituents are in a constant dance of to-and-fro, in-and-out, come-and-go. We have high tides and low tides, sunny days and rainy days, inflation and recession. All things in existence, including existence itself, is in a constant state of flux and transformation.

When we look at our body, it appears static and permanent, yet it is constantly in a state of transformation through an eternal dance of exchange with the rest of the world. Our body, which looks solid, is actually composed of trillions of cells and millions of trillions of atoms and molecules. These atoms, molecules, and cells are constantly changing and transforming.

Everything in our body is in constant exchange with the rest of the environment. We breathe in air from the outside atmosphere and breathe out air from our lungs. We take in food through our mouth and we eliminate the waste. The cells of our body are constantly being replaced by new cells. The only reason we experience long-term chronic illness is because our bodies reconstruct that illness. The body replaces diseased cells which have died off with new diseased cells. In truth, those diseased cells are just as new as the healthy cells that have recently been created. Every year, every cell, tissue, and organ in your body has been replaced, sometimes multiple times. We are constantly being renewed. Nothing is the same at any moment. With this understanding, we can begin to watch as our inner potential unfolds. We can participate in our ever-evolving selves, rather than allowing it to happen by default. Knowing that our bodies are ever-changing, and that every effect has a cause, we can begin to consciously decide what we want our body to become (the effect) and begin taking the appropriate steps (the cause) in order to create our desired intention (a healthy body).

Change is inevitable. The only choice we have is whether to grow or to decay.

HEALING PRINCIPLE #4

The Law of Inclusive Evolution

The *law of inclusive evolution* states that the whole is always greater than the sum of its parts, and that all things that are individual are always a part of something greater, including ourselves. When we look at how our physical world is created, its design is apparent as a system of smaller, lesser parts making up larger, more complex wholes. Very often, these larger wholes are actually parts of even larger wholes, ad infinitum.

Ken Wilber, author of such works as *A Brief History of Everything* and *The Marriage of Sense and Soul*, calls this concept *nesting*. Atoms are nested into molecules, which are nested into more and more complex organic structures all the way up to the highest functions of the human brain and nervous system. Each level incorporates all the ones before it, adding to each new level more evolved qualities and functions.[3]

Everything has its building blocks. Yet, when two things merge to form something else, that something always functions on a higher level. Everything is greater than the sum of its parts. When you take two atoms of hydrogen, (a gas), and you mix it with one atom of oxygen, (also a gas), you get neither a gas nor anything which resembles either hydrogen or oxygen, you get a liquid – *water*.

If you put hydrogen, carbon, nitrogen and oxygen together in certain configurations you acquire different molecules in the form of proteins, carbohydrates, and fats. Depending how these molecules are configured will determine the type of living cell that is created – bacteria, animal, or plant. Organizing the cells into synergistic families creates tissues and organs, together manifesting a living, breathing organism.

Although a human brain is more complex than the cells that comprise it, and the cells are more complex than the atoms that make it up, there can be no cell without atoms and there can be no brain without cells.

Whereas the atom does not hold within itself the qualities of the cell, and the cell does not hold the properties of the brain, when two or more individuals come together and work synergistically, something greater results, that is more efficient, more complex and more evolved.

Through this harmonious interaction of the smaller, constituent parts, the more evolved whole is manifested. Evolution is the process by which something becomes more: more complex, more integrated, more efficient, more organized, or more intelligent. Our universe and all of its parts are in an eternal process of evolution. This process is not one of greater individuality, as has been taught through the schools of Darwinian evolution and survival of the fittest, instead, it is one of greater harmony, greater awareness, and greater efficiency.

Everything in nature moves toward three qualities: greater harmony, awareness, and efficiency. Whether we watch water move into an empty space or a family of chimpanzees communing in the jungle, we will observe this notion. While this process does take time, we can experience it by observing how we develop as individuals.

At some moment in your past, two cells, a sperm and an egg, came together. Before their meeting, they were individual, separate entities with completely different properties and qualities. With their uniting, a new cell was created. This cell not only possessed both the qualities of the sperm and the qualities of the egg, it possessed newer more complex qualities. In their union, they became something more ... a cell with the ability to grow and develop into a living, breathing, thinking, and feeling human being – a quality that both the sperm and egg lacked. In their harmonious interaction, they became something more – they evolved.

In becoming human beings over the last 4.5 billion years that life has been on this planet, life has passed through progressively more advanced, more adaptive, and more intelligent stages of life – from one-celled bacteria to multi-cellular organisms such as amoebae to sea-creatures such as sea-cucumbers and jellyfish. From there, animals began to develop spines and are called vertebrates. These vertebrates evolved from fish to amphibians such as frogs and salamanders to reptiles such as snakes and lizards to birds and finally to mammals from which we evolved.

As life passed through each stage of evolution, not only did it retain the qualities of the creatures from which it evolved, but it acquired new, more advanced qualities. This is what is meant by inclusive evolution – new generations evolving to more advanced states while including the properties of their less evolved ancestors.

For example, in passing through the various stages of fish, reptile, and mammal, we acquired the physical traits and neural characteristics of these animals. From the early invertebrates and insects, we attained the basic necessities of life: respiration, digestion, reproduction and other vital functions. Through the fish and reptile, we began to experience desire, the inner drive for survival of both ourselves and our species. We obtained the inner experience of hunger – for food, water, and sex. The fight or flight mechanism went into full force and every nerve of our being began to strive for sustenance and longevity.

As we began to emerge into the stage of mammal, some of our greatest gifts were achieved. It is through this stage that we began to care for another, learning to interact in family units and tribal communities. We began to nurture and mother our young. We began to hunt and rest with our brethren. We began to feel the pulse of emotion and spend time in activities of play. Finally, we evolved to human being, capable of thought, creativity and reason.

In analyzing the concept of evolution, a common question arose in the scientific community: Where does evolution take place? For a while it was believed that evolution occurred during the life of the animal. For example, there was once a creature that stretched its neck to reach for fruit high in a tree. Over time, with consistent effort, its neck began to stretch. When this creature had offspring, these offspring had long necks and we had our first giraffes. After genetics was discovered and DNA realized, we began to understand that evolution does not occur outside amongst the trees and valleys, but within the genetic matrix of our cells.

According to this theory, mutations, or random changes, in our genetic structure is what causes evolution. Those random changes that were not in the best interest of the organism, either had no effect or caused the organism to die. However, if the change allowed the organism to survive longer and easier, it was retained in the genetic matrix and passed on to its offspring. The creature had evolved.

According to cell biologist and genetic physicist Bruce Lipton, both theories are correct. Dr. Lipton's theory states that although the evolutionary changes do occur within our genetic structure, they are influenced by our environment and our perception of the environment. Based upon his research at Stanford University, Dr. Lipton has shown that cell behavior and genetic evolution are influenced by consciousness. He has shown that "the membranes of the cell can actually influence genetic structure, and that cell membrane behavior is influenced by consciousness and our perception of the environment. Cells actually have the ability to rewrite their DNA when environmentally prompted. This rewriting is typically positively adaptive and most likely accounts for 95-98% of all evolutionary change." [4]

Watching the development of the human child, embryologists (scientists who study pre-natal development of fetuses, embryos, and infants) began to realize that as a human child develops in the womb, it passes through stages in which it physically resembles the embryos of less evolved organisms, such as birds, reptiles, or dogs. And, as they pass through these developmental stages, they take on the characteristics of that animal. Watching this process they concluded: Evolution takes place within every womb of every expectant mother throughout the natural world.

Once the sperm and egg come together to form the single cell, it embarks on a journey of inclusive evolution, passing through each stage of animal evolution that has occurred upon this planet.

Through a nine-month process of transformation and development, it passes through stages in which it resembles fish, bird, reptile, early mammal, such as a dog, and primate, taking on the characteristics of each phase and evolving to the next, eventually developing into a perfect little human being, capable of logic and reason. Able to reflect on the past and envision the future. Gifted with the faculties of imagination and creativity, we can begin choosing thought and developing our lives and our environment according to our desire. We are the culmination of everything that has come before. This is the meaning of *inclusive evolution*, to incorporate the lesser to become something greater.

In summary, all things are made up of smaller parts, and all things are greater than the sum of its parts. Why is it important for us to understand this concept on our clear path to healing? It is important for two reasons: to appreciate your parts and to appreciate your part.

First, to appreciate your parts. Quite often, when we become sick or injured, we tend to alienate that part of us. When we look at something as a part, it becomes apart – separate. The part that is already damaged, sick, or separated is communicating with you, through pain, disease, and discomfort. Like a fallen child that has chafed his or her knee, this damaged part is calling for your loving attention. It wants to be part of the whole, yet what do we do? We say things like, "my bad knee," "my knee is killing me," and "I wish it would just go away." Then we take medications to numb the pain, that alienate the part even more. And, if all else fails, we remove the part.

What the healing principle of inclusive evolution tells us, is that only by including the part into the family of the whole, can true healing take place. When we allow ourselves to feel the pain of the alienated and diseased part and welcome it back, only then we will experience wholeness and healing. If we found our child screaming with an injured knee, we would not put a bandage over his or her mouth to stop the screaming. We do precisely that, when it comes to our own health, by taking medicines to make the symptoms and pains go away.

What should we do? We should nurture the child and fulfill all the child's needs. If we are truly to heal, we must appreciate our parts and treat them as we would a child – hold them, nurture them, love them.

To fully appreciate our parts and understand the importance of this healing principle, there is another aspect that must be addressed, and that is to appreciate *our part*. Just as each of our cells and body parts contribute to make up who we are, you are also like a cell within the greater body of our planet Earth. Just as our body can not exist without each and every cell that composes it, our human family can not exist without you.

Each of us is a vital component of something much greater, much more complex, and much more evolved. Each of us has something to contribute that adds to the greater wholeness of our world. Just as our bodies become sick through the dis-ease of the individual cells, so does our world suffer when one of us suffers. When we appreciate our important part in the health and wholeness of the world, we begin to reclaim our individual power and accept the responsibility to heal ourselves. It is only through the healing of ourselves will we heal the world.

When we understand the healing principle of inclusive evolution, we begin to appreciate the complexity of ourselves and the world around us. We then acknowledge the important part each of us plays in this grand universe and the importance of every cell, molecule, and atom. Looking at the world around us with this new insight, we become aware of the complex organization of which every pebble possesses, never mind the dynamic web of interactive chemical reactions within the human body or the infinite weaving of neurons within the human brain.

Witnessing the wonder of this universe and its harmonious organization and orchestration, a new question starts to emerge within the observing mind: What causes the organizing and orchestrating?

HEALING PRINCIPLE #5

The Law of Universal Intelligence

In observing the world, it is not difficult to surmise that there is an order to things. When you watch the workings of nature and the universe, it becomes apparent that there exists certain principles or laws that govern things.

It is difficult to argue that if you plant an apple seed, and it germinates, the result will always be an apple tree. Just as an apple seed always produces an apple tree, there are a multitude of laws and principles that govern the workings within the universe. What is not so obvious is from where did these rules come? What dictates that this is the way things should be?

To answer this question, it is difficult not to deviate from the realm of science into the realm of metaphysics or spirituality, yet even in the scientific community only one answer could be surmised and it is this: There is a Universal Intelligence within all things that maintains them in existence, gives to them all their properties, and governs their behavior.

We live in an intelligent universe. According to *Webster*, the definition of intelligent is "a) the ability to know and learn, b) the ability to cope with a new situation, c) to possess information."[5]

Earlier we came to realize that all matter in its truest form is, in fact, bundles of energy. We also came to understand that all energy is vibration. Inherent in all energy and vibration is *information*. That is why our eyes, ears, and other sense organs are able to experience the world, by interpreting the information inherent in vibration. If all matter is energy and vibration, and all vibration carries within it information, then all things in the universe possess information.

Yet, does this make the universe intelligent? A book contains information, but is it intelligent? It is not enough to possess information. There must be something more. It must have awareness. It must be able to experience itself and influence its own expression. According to *Webster*, it must be able to know and learn and be able to cope with new situations. It must have the ability to evolve, change and transform itself into higher levels of creativity, abstraction, and unpredictability, what Dr. Deepak Chopra calls "the hallmarks of intelligence."[6]

Do we see evidence of this in the world around us? Do we see a universe that learns, grows, and evolves? Absolutely. From the bees that fly around our heads, to the plants that sprout from the ground, to the stars and galaxies that are ever shining above our heads, we witness an ever-changing, ever-evolving world. Every day, as they observe our world, scientists, specifically the physicists and astronomers, are realizing the intelligent nature of our universe. They have even named this the *Unified Field*.[7] This unified field is the field of intelligence where all energy originates and from where the natural laws that govern this universe reside. It is this intelligence that gives to all things their qualities, properties, and patterns of behavior. It is this intelligence that gives to matter the ability to inclusively evolve as described in the last healing principle. It is this property that gives to matter the ability to be something greater than the sum of its parts.

It is not difficult to view an animal or plant as possessing intelligence, but it becomes difficult when we look at a rock or a flame. Yet these too possess intelligence ... at a different level of awareness. With each level of awareness comes the increased ability to interact with the environment. A rock has one level of awareness, giving it the ability to maintain its existence and react with other substances to form new rocks. A plant, has a greater level of awareness, giving it additional abilities to respond to sunlight and water. It grows and changes with the seasons. It reproduces and interacts with other plants. It has a higher level of awareness and intelligence than the rock. Animals have advanced one step further allowing them to feel and communicate. They interact in groups and families. They can strategize and influence their environment with purpose and reason, culminating with the most aware and intelligent – the human being.

When we look at a living thing, what does it possess that a non-living thing does not?

A living thing possesses greater levels of awareness and intelligence. It is more organized and requires greater degrees of orchestration. It has the ability to self-reflect, to observe and adjust itself in relation to the environment around it. It is this special quality of adaptability that causes a living thing to grow under stress, while an inanimate object, such as a broom, wears away under similar forces. It is this special quality of intelligence – depending on its degree of self-awareness – that gives life to the living. It is this vitalistic principle that allows human beings to continuously grow, evolve, and heal.

In the last section, we discussed the beautiful interaction of the sperm and egg, and their union to become something much greater – the beginning of a human life. This singular cell is the genesis of a lifetime of joy and tribulation, love and grief, accomplishments and failures. It is perfect in its singularity. Within it, is a marvelous structure of energy, information, and intelligence – the DNA molecule.

The DNA molecule is the culmination of all the intelligence that ever existed. This molecule contains the information to manifest the greatest creation in all the universe, the human being. It holds the blueprint of every cell, organ, and chemical reaction within the human body. It possesses the data for the shape and function of every organ and tissue, and the method by which all the constituent parts of the human body should interact. We've discovered that within this tiny structure lies the secret of personality, desire, and consciousness.

After a few hours of being created, something miraculous happens to this single cell – it divides. It produces an exact duplicate of itself, of which also carries the DNA molecule in its entirety, so that we have two exact replicas of the germinal cell of human creation. These cells divide again and again to produce four cells ... then eight ... sixteen ... thirty-two ... sixty-four ... one hundred twenty eight and so on, producing a round sphere of conglomerate cells each of which is an exact replica of all the others. Each of these many cells has the exact same instructional molecule within it, the genetic matrix of the DNA molecule.

Although each of these cells are exactly alike, each containing the same genetic material as all the others, around the second to third week after fertilization, something miraculous begins to happen. At this time, a process known as differentiation begins to take place. One of the cells "raises its hand" and proclaims, "I am going to become a nerve cell," and it begins to change its shape and function until it becomes a nerve cell, capable of transmitting impulses of energy and information. Another cell says, "I am going to be a heart cell," and it begins to differentiate, changing its shape and function to become a heart cell, capable of keeping a rhythmic beat. Another becomes a liver cell, and a skin cell, and a bone cell, and so on. Each cell completely different in shape and function from all the others, until between weeks four and eight, a tiny human embryo develops.

This is a miraculous process. That two cells can come together, share some information, and unite to eventually develop into a fully functioning human being is a miracle of nature. Yet the truest miracle is not immediately apparent. Before differentiation, all the cells are exactly the same, each carrying the same genetic instructions. If they are all exactly the same, carrying the same instructions, how did one cell *know* to become a nerve cell and another know to become a liver cell? How did one cell know to read "Chapter 28" of the DNA molecule to become a heart cell and another know to read "Chapter 4" on how to become bone? They all had the same instructions, yet how did they know what to differentiate into? How did they decide who would become what? Throughout all science and biological research and development, throughout the centuries, only one answer has been found and it is – *they just know!*

There is an intelligence within all living cells that cannot be seen, measured, or analyzed. It is the information within the vibration within the energy within all matter. It is a knowing that is not within the genetic code but within the matrix of the substance of matter. Those cells knew to differentiate, not because the genetic material told them to, they differentiated because they are intelligent. A blueprint does not construct the house, it requires an architect to read the instructions and build it. So do the cells read the genetic code, interpret it, and build a human being. All the cells of the body are inherently intelligent. There is an innate intelligence within all living things that coordinates their existence, orchestrates their living systems, and heals their wounds.

If the cells are able to read the genetic material and form themselves and the body by interpreting its instruction, who or what was the architect that designed the complex blueprints of the genetic material to begin with? There is only one answer. There is a *universal intelligence* within all things that maintains them in existence and gives to them all properties and qualities.

With the understanding and appreciation of this intelligence within all things, we begin to see the world in a new way, especially the physical body we presently call home. With this knowledge, there are only "on purpose's," never accidents. Everything our body does, whether it's the experience of orgasm or suffering, is an intelligent response. There is no such thing as malfunction, disorder or disease, only intelligent adaptations, changes, and transformations in response to changes in our environment.

HEALING PRINCIPLE #6

The Law of Unified Abundance

The *law of unified abundance* states that all things are one, however, this unified essence manifests as a collective abundance of individuated parts, that are in and of themselves, one. It is a one and many universe.

Our universe is one vibration. Everything that exists, physical and non-physical, are manifestations of vibration. There appears to be separation among all the various entities that exist in the universe, yet, they are all manifestations of *one* vibration.

Our reality is nothing but an interconnected web of energetic interactions and vibrational expressions. Just as the ocean is a united body of water forever expressing waves throughout its being, so is the universe a united ocean of energy forever expressing vibration throughout itself. In fact, the word abundance is a latin term which means "to ride away in waves."

We look at the world and each other and it appears that I am separate from you and you are separate from me. We appear separate from the trees that are separate from the sky above and its infinitude of stars. Yet, this is an illusion of our senses. If we saw things as they truly are rather than through our five senses, we would see an ocean of vibration and energy that is never-ending, infinitely whole and contiguous. Where we would usually see a solid object such as a table or a person, instead you would see an increased density or a thicker glob of energy. The borders of such objects would fade into less dense matter to once again coalesce into the next object.

The air that you are breathing right now is not separate from the air in the next room. It is contiguous with the air outside your residence and continues into the next city, state, and country. Air that encompasses the entire planet, blends with space beyond our atmosphere out into the cosmos. The energy and vibration that is within and is all things, is just like the air. It is continuous throughout all physical and non-physical things, making up all material objects, all electromagnetism, all thoughts, feelings, and if you are so inclined, spirit.

When we understand the interconnected oneness of things, we begin to appreciate the interconnectedness of our cells, organs, and body functions. When we hurt our arm, it is not an injury to our arm, but to our whole being. When we have a sore throat, it is not an encapsulated problem within the throat but an adaptive change in which the entire body is involved. When we experience pain of any kind, this is a signal that a part has lost its perception of connectiveness with the rest of the body. It has become alienated, lost, separated, or disconnected. It is very common to further alienate or disconnect that part by numbing it with medication or even worse removing it altogether through surgery. Healing is the process of becoming whole, of reuniting all separate parts into a once-again cohesive whole.

These concepts are not restricted to our personal experience and the healing of our individual selves, but extend into our communities and the world around us. As previously discussed in chapter 3, in the sixth cause of the health-care crisis, it is this concept of separation that produces the diseases and ills of our society: crime, drug abuse, and hatred.

Only through the experience of separateness and the perception of "other" are these things possible. If each of us were to see the other as a manifestation and expression of ourselves, these things would not be possible. Criminal punishment, finger-pointing, and blame only produces further separation, perpetuating these ills of our society. Only through the perception of oneness and unity, otherwise known as Love, can the diseases of our society be truly healed. If the truth is that all things are always connected, then the experience of separateness is an illusion of perception.

The most important aspect of healing is our perception of the world around us. When we alter our perception and our system of beliefs to one in alignment with healing and the true nature of our universe, we then experience the wholeness within us, the truest essence of who we are, and we express our dearest unique gifts with the rest of the world.

When we begin to change our perceptions and belief systems, we see the world change. We see things in a new way, and see things we never saw before. Experiencing these changes in our world, we realize that the world dances to our every whim and we understand it is merely a manifestation of our thoughts.

Let's look at the *law of subjective creation*, and discover how this last healing principle is actually the source of all the others.

HEALING PRINCIPLE #7

The Law of Subjective Creation

The *law of subjective creation* states that everything that exists within the outside, objective, physical world is a manifestation of our personal, subjective thought. When we tie together the previous six principles, this idea becomes self-evident.

Everything that exists is merely the effect of a previously expressed cause. Both cause and effect are expressions of energy and vibration that are in a constant state of change. This change is not haphazard, but in a constant process of transformation, growth, and evolution, uniting all individual parts into more complex systems of organization. This process is orchestrated by an infinite intelligence that is universal in scope, maintaining all things in existence and giving to them, their properties and functions. As manifestations of one vibration and the expression of one intelligence, all things in existence are in essence united as one.

If we accept this as true – as demonstrated through both logic and scientific reason, as well as by personal experimentation through life experience – we come to realize this last universal principle: that all things in existence are the expression of one intelligence, one mind. That the world around us is the objective experience of a subjective idea.

The idea that our thoughts create our reality is more than just a metaphysical, spiritual teaching, it is an actual statement of neuroscience. As discussed earlier, our experience of the world comes to us through our five senses. How we experience the world is determined by our brain and nervous system. Our past experiences and neurological tone determine how our brain interprets the data coming in through our senses. For example, if as a child I was attacked by a bear while walking through the woods, as an adult, I would have a different experience walking through the woods compared to my friend who made love to his first girlfriend in the forest. We would both experience a walk through the woods, but our perception of the experience would be entirely different – one of fear, one of love.

Everything we perceive and bring into our nervous system via our senses, passes through filters produced by past experiences, belief systems, and our *neurological tone*. Neurological tone is the actual physical level of tension present in our nerve tissue. Similar to how a guitar string produces different notes when tightened to different levels of tension, we experience the world differently when our nerves are in different levels of tension. The ideal tone of our nerves is one of ease. Due to various physical, emotional, and chemical stresses that influence us every day, the tension in our neural tissue can be altered, sometimes causing dis-ease.

To experience this, let's do an experiment with posture. First, sit in a chair. Allow your head to hang down and let your shoulders slump forward. Place your hands between your knees and place your feet flat on the floor beneath you. How do you feel? Notice your breathing. Is it full and deep or shallow and short? Try to laugh. Is it difficult or easy? This is the posture of dis-ease. It actually increases the level of tension in your spinal cord and nerves. This is the posture of depression and illness. In this posture it is almost impossible to experience joy and health, but easy to experience sorrow and illness.

Now, let us change our posture and change the neurological tone. Sit up. Lift your chin towards the ceiling. Bring your hands and arms up and out. Extend your feet and legs out in front of you and slightly arch your back. How do you feel? I can imagine that immediately you took a deep breath and a smile appeared across your face. This posture reduces the level of tension in your spine and nervous system, putting you into a posture of ease and well-being. Change the posture, change the tone – change your experience and perception of the world around you. Did the world change? No. But your thoughts about the world did, which created a new world around you. Whether the actual world changed or your belief that the world changed does not matter. In your experience, it has changed. Your thought created your reality.

When you learn to use this process consciously with purpose and intention, all of your dreams, desires, and goals will be created before you, producing a *Garden of Eden* of your own creation.

1.   Wattles, Wallace, *The Science of Getting Rich*, 1902,
2.   Robbins, Anthony, *Awaken the Giant Within*, Fireside, 1993, p. 82.
3.   Wilber, Ken, *The Marriage of Sense and Soul*, Random House, 1996, pp. 6-11.
4.   Lipton, Bruce, Ph.D, "Cell Biology and the Science of Innate Intelligence."
5.   *Webster's Seventh New Collegiate Dictionary*, G.&C. Merrium Co., 1965, p. 440.
6.   Chopra, Deepak, M.D., Simon, David, M.D., *Training the Mind, Healing the Body*, Audiocassettes, Nightingale-Conant, 1997.
7.   Capra, Frijof, *The Tao of Physics*, Shambala, 1991.

A New Vision of Truth : Summary

There are seven principles that govern how everything in the universe functions, including health and healing. These principles are:

1. **The Law of Cause and Effect** – Everything in existence has a cause and an effect on everything else.
2. **The Law of Energy and Vibration** – Everything in the universe is in its truest essence pure energy and is in a constant state of movement and vibration.
3. **The Law of Perpetual Change** – Everything in the universe is in a constant state of change and transformation.
4. **The Law of Inclusive Evolution** – The whole is always greater than the sum of its parts; and all things that are individual are always a part of something greater.
5. **The Law of Universal Intelligence** – There is a Universal Intelligence within all things that maintains them in existence, gives them their properties, and governs their behavior.
6. **The Law of Unified Abundance** – It is a one and many universe. All things are one, yet, this unified essence manifests as a collective abundance of individuated parts that are of themselves, one.
7. **The Law of Subjective Creation** – The outside world is a reflection of our inner thoughts, feelings, and beliefs.

6

THE SEVEN ATTRIBUTES OF HEALTH
The Seven Response Abilities

The natural healing force within us is the greatest force in getting well.
~ Hippocrates, the Father of Medicine

What is this thing we all desire? What is this quality called Health we all seek? What does it mean to be Healthy and what does it mean to Heal? Often when I ask these questions, the answers I get are: "To feel good," "To be free of disease," and, "To not be sick." There is a common perception that health is merely a state of feeling good and not having disease. Yet, the World Health Organization defines Health as "complete physical, emotional, mental, and social well-being, and not merely the absence of disease or infirmity."[1]

The word "Health" and its root "Heal" come from an old English word "hal" that means whole.[2] Health, therefore, is a state of wholeness, and to heal is to become whole. Health is the state of all the different parts working in harmony as one. You are healthy when all of you is functioning at peak efficiency and performance.

Why is it that the common understanding of health is limited to *no disease* and *feeling good*, when its definition is so much broader? Health encompasses the experience of our body, emotions, mind, relationships, society, and finances. It consists of balance, harmony, and well-being. Somehow the meaning of health has been reduced to something comparable to numbness, in which feeling is avoided and our fullest expression is condemned. In this chapter, you will learn that healing only occurs when we allow ourselves to feel completely and express ourselves to our fullest potential.

Working as a healing facilitator, assisting people to reach higher levels of health and wellness, as well as studying health, philosophy, psychology, world history, spiritual matters, and success, I have found there are seven common attributes throughout all of these areas which define Health. Whether it is the health of the human body, the mind, the emotions, a family, finances, a relationship, a corporation, a nation, or a world, each of these seven attributes must be present. These seven attributes are different abilities by which we respond to our environment. I call them the seven *Response Abilities*. They are:

1. The response ability to *perceive* change.
2. The response ability to *adapt* to change.
3. The response ability to *recover* from an adaptation to change.
4. The response ability to *grow and evolve*.
5. The response ability to *express* physically a mental or emotional intention.
6. The response ability to *harmoniously interact* with others.
7. The response ability to experience *contentment*.

Health is the state in which any whole, and all of its parts, have these seven response abilities functioning at their optimum potential. This whole may be a human cell; an organ, such as the heart; an organ system, such as the digestive system; or the entire body. This whole might be the human mind or emotional body. It may be our finances, relationships, or career. Or it might be a family, a community, a nation, a world, possibly the entire universe. In order to have health, all seven attributes must be present.

Healing is the process of increasing or regaining Health. It is the path by which one regains one or all of these seven qualities that may have been lost, or the process by which one of these seven qualities becomes more effective, more efficient, and more sensitive. However, if one is lost, all the others suffer. For instance, if we lose our ability to perceive change, we are unable to adapt, thereby losing our ability to grow and evolve. On the other hand, if one of these attributes is healed, they are all healed. They are seven separate qualities acting as one experience ... optimum health.

Let us look at each *response ability* and then we will examine how they work together.

RESPONSE ABILITY #1

Perception

The winds of change are ever-blowing. All around us life and its environment are in constant interaction. We can define the environment as those factors that influence life; the air we breathe, the food we eat, the ground which we walk on, the people we meet, are all examples of our environment – our external environment.

We also have an internal environment. Within us is a vast landscape teetering on a tender balance of temperature, pressure, and an infinitely complex system of chemical exchange. These factors within us maintain life, such as body temperature; blood pressure; salt, sugar, and other chemical levels; as well as our thoughts, emotions, beliefs, and intentions.

Environmental factors, internal and external, are not static. They are in a constant state of change rising and falling, ebbing and flowing. In order to survive the eternal cycle of change, we must be aware that a change has been made. We must perceive the change, either through our five senses or through other internal senses such as proprioception (the ability to sense our position in space), nociception (the ability to detect pain), baroception (the ability to detect pressure changes), and thermoception (the ability to detect temperature changes).[3]

These environmental changes can be very subtle, and out of the range of our physical senses. In these instances, more subtle perceptions may be experienced, such as intuition, "gut" feelings, sudden insights, synchronicity, meaningful coincidences, premonition, and prophecy.

We mentioned earlier that the primary principle of healing is that every cause has an effect and every effect has its cause. In physics, this is described as every action having an equal and opposite reaction. This in the world of nature and living things is called *stimulus* and *response*.

All of life and its functions are based on the principle of stimulus and response. That is when there is a change in the environment, whether internal or external, of which the organism becomes aware and responds to. For example, the organism may become aware of or perceive a deficiency of nutrients as an experience of hunger, of which he responds to by looking for and ingesting some form of food. These changes are as subtle as a slight change in temperature or pressure or as dramatic as hearing the roar of a lion behind your back, either way it requires a response.

In order for there to be a response, change must be perceived. If we are not aware of a change in the environment, we can not respond to it. This can be very dangerous. If we do not feel the heat of the fire, we can not pull our hand away and protect ourselves from being burned.

Our bodies are equipped with tiny receptors that monitor every change in chemistry, pressure, and temperature. Similar to the thermostat in the house that keeps the room temperature at a predetermined level of comfort, our receptors maintain the delicate balance of our body's subtle chemistry and biomechanics. If we do not perceive the slight changes that alter the delicate balance of our biochemistry, we can die instantly.

The more subtle and sensitive we can perceive changes in our inner and outer environment, the more readily and efficiently we can make the necessary response. Would you rather hear the roar of the lion miles away, or feel its breath upon your neck? Would you rather feel the subtle signal of the body telling you there needs to be a change in your diet or exercise, or wait until you are in a crisis ten to twenty years later being rushed to the hospital with a coronary arrest. The more subtle and sensitive our ability to perceive change, the greater our ability to achieve our optimum healing potential.

To have health, we must have the ability to *perceive* changes in our environment. But once perceived, we must be able to adjust in accordance with change. We must be able to adapt.

RESPONSE ABILITY #2

Adaptation

Ancient Chinese wisdom says that when the wind blows strong, the mighty oak which stands firm, will topple, yet the flowing reeds will live to see another day. Likewise, when we experience change, we must be able to adapt, we must "go with the flow." If we stand firm, resisting change, like the mighty oak, we will fall. If instead, we bend like the gentle reed, we will live to see another day, becoming stronger and wiser in the process.

Our bodies have a remarkable ability to *adapt* to change – to change itself internally to best survive a change on the outside, receiving the fullest benefit from the experience. Left on its own, the human body can survive tremendous trial and tribulation because of its wonderful adaptive mechanism. Infants who usually would be considered unfit to care for themselves, have been found lost in the woods or trapped in a well, alive and thriving after days, and even weeks, without food and water. Although these conditions are not optimum for the health and well-being of a child, the child's resilience and adaptability is demonstrated in such situations.

The most primitive and best known example of the human adaptive mechanism is the fight or flight response. This unconscious animal response occurs when we are placed in danger. The body automatically prepares itself for one of two adaptive responses – to either confront the danger or run away. Civilization has eliminated much of our need for this response, yet it still stands and protects us in times of physical challenge or emotional contention.

When this type of situation arises, a number of internal adaptations occur. Our adrenal glands release adrenaline into our blood stream giving us a burst of energy. Our digestive system slows or stops completely to reserve energy resources. Our eyes dilate, pupils open wide so that we can see more in less light. Our blood pressure and pulse rate increase sending more blood and oxygen to all the cells of our body, especially the muscles. All these responses are created in order to prepare us for action and increase our chances of survival in a challenging situation.

In the past our adaptive mechanism was responsible in determining whether we survived a given situation. Today however, this mechanism may even perform the same function, but due to our development of civilization, society and culture, these responses to change hold a more subtle, yet profound, function, one that allows us to get the most out of any situation, especially in the areas of healing, growth, and further evolution of our species.

If we adapt to a change in the environment and become stronger, smarter, or more sensitive, we will become more advanced as a species and achieve higher levels of awareness, accomplishment, and healing.

To reach our highest levels of health and healing, we must ensure that our bodies and minds are capable of effective and efficient adaptation to change in the environment. With more sensitivity and perception, we are better prepared and forewarned to make necessary changes. If this Response Ability to adapt or change ourselves in relationship to the outside environment is not functioning at its peak, perception is futile. If we were to perceive a possible danger and were unable to respond to it, what use is the perception? It is like a starving man looking across a great cavern at an apple tree with no way of reaching it. Unless we adapt effectively to the changes that we have perceived, the perception holds no purpose and serves only to frustrate.

Understanding the important function of perception and adaptation, let us look at the next response ability ... the ability to *recover*.

RESPONSE ABILITY #3

Recovery

The wind blows. The reed bends into the wind. Yet, what happens when the wind stops blowing? The reed returns to its original position, standing strong, pointing up towards the sun. The reed *recovers*. If the wind was stronger than the reed's ability to adapt and recover appropriately, the reed would break and remain in its bent position. In order for the reed to maintain its health, it must be able to perceive the stress of the wind, adapt to the stress and then recover from the adaptation.

Like the reed, we must recover from any adaptation we experience due to change, once the conditions return to normal. Many of our adaptations are temporary changes to best survive the "passing storm." Using the fight or flight response as an example, once the danger passes, the blood pressure, pulse rate, and adrenaline levels must return to a resting state. The digestive system must proceed with its vital activity and our dilated pupils need to return to normal size. In other words, the body has to recover from the event.

Other factors of the body, such as temperature, pressure, and a multitude of chemical reactions, are in a continuous, never-ending balancing act. For example, insulin is the hormone that controls the glucose (blood sugar) level in our blood. Ultimately, it is glucose that provides fuel for the body, especially the brain. When we eat something that contains sugar or starch, insulin is released by the pancreas into the blood stream to remove excess sugar from the blood and store it for later use. Once the sugar level is within optimum levels, the insulin level in the blood is reduced. If there is not enough sugar in the blood, a counter-hormone called glucagon is released that draws sugar from reserves and releases it into the blood stream to provide energy for the body. This see-saw effect of insulin and glucagon is just one example of millions of such balancing acts that occur in the body.[4]

What would happen, if once the blood sugar level reached its optimum level, the pancreas continued to release insulin? Because of this lack of recovery, more sugar would be removed from the blood than was necessary producing a "condition" called hypoglycemia or low blood sugar. What if, after an intense physical or emotional crisis, the necessary increase in blood pressure and adrenaline never returned to states of rest? This lack of recovery would result in anxiety and hypertension or high blood pressure. If during a state of repair, the mechanism that holds the normal rate of cell division and reproduction in check, failed to do its job what would happen? This lack of recovery would result in cancer. As you can see, many of our long-term chronic illnesses are nothing more than a normal response to change, or adaptation, that never recovered once the change had passed.

When looking at diseases, conditions, and illnesses diagnosed by mankind, you will find that *all* of them are caused by either a failure to perceive change in the inner or outer environment, a failure to effectively adapt to the change, or a failure to recover once the change had passed. This might be an overnight process or it could take many years, decades or even an entire lifetime. All the circumstances, experiences and events that effect the body, mind and nervous system, contribute to increased dysfunction and disease, if we don't respond appropriately.

When looking at any disease process, rarely is it caused by one thing. There are often many physical, emotional, and mental factors that influence the body and contribute to our health and our disease. On this clear path to healing, we address health on all levels to assist the body and mind to regain, improve, and develop their ability to perceive, adapt, and recover to change – its *response ability*.

This process of recovery is effective in returning the body back to its previous state before the adaptation took place, once a given change is no longer present in the environment. However, what happens if the environmental conditions do not return to normal and the change does not go away? What if the wind continues to blow? What if a new environment is created in which the adaptation must become permanent in order to survive? In that case, recovery is not necessary, but *evolution* is.

RESPONSE ABILITY #4

Evolution

When the winds of change blow, they can change the landscape of our environment. Sand and soil may be pushed into hills, and over time, mountains. Rivers may be redirected, and lakes may, over time, form. Although the wind may stop blowing, its effects have created a lasting impression. In such conditions, there are two choices: to grow or to decay. Living things, such as trees, animals, and people, grow and evolve. Inert, non-living things, such as stones and sticks, decay. Wash running water over a seed and watch what happens ... it grows. Wash running water over a stone and what happens? It erodes.

Growth and evolution is a continual process of change by which a simple state or condition is transformed into a higher, more complex state. A healthy body or any other organization always allows for change to cause growth and evolution. On the other hand, an *unhealthy* body decays and eventually ceases to exist.

Evolution and growth is nothing more than a long-term adaptive response. An example of this would be the experience of muscle building as a result of weight training. The act of lifting heavy weights over and over is actually perceived by the body as a danger or crisis. These weights place stress on the muscles, bones, ligaments, and joints. In order to protect itself, the body builds more muscle tissue in order to prepare itself for future experiences of such stress. If we continue to work out regularly, increasing the weight as we get stronger, this process will continue indefinitely.

What differs in this situation from the previously mentioned adaptive response, is the body is now stronger, more effective, and more efficient even after the stress is gone. Recognizing this, theoretically, the body says, "I am stronger, more effective, and more efficient as a result of this adaptation ... this one's a keeper."

Another example of evolution and growth would be that of sun-tanning. The darkening of the skin as a result of laying in the sun is a healthy response of the body producing more melanin in the skin. Melanin is a pigmented protein that protects the skin from the damaging effects of ultraviolet radiation. Tanning is caused not by the sun's rays, but by an adaptation produced by the body in response to the exposure of ultraviolet light. If the exposure to sunlight is continuous and frequent like muscle building, this adaptation will become permanent.

Since the response ability of adaptation is necessary to protect us from sudden changes that may be damaging, even deadly, the *response ability of evolution* – though not as urgent – is necessary for the long-term survival of our species, and life in general on our planet. Through this ability we are to learn from our experiences and become stronger, wiser, and more effective as a species. This process is perpetual and is responsible for our human family moving from the primitive existence as an ape to the spiritual and intellectual wonder we are today. In this infinite arena we call our universe, we are yet at the beginning of our evolutionary experience.

RESPONSE ABILITY #5

Expression

When the wind blows across the land, sometimes it carries with it seeds. What is a seed? A seed is nothing more than an intention. Look inside an acorn. Do you find a little oak tree? What you find is dust. Yet, within that dust is the information and intention that, with the right conditions, will produce the mighty oak. In other words, what separates an acorn from a stone, is its ability to express physically, a non-physical or intelligent intention.

In any body, organization, or situation, the ability to express physically a mental or emotional intention is necessary to be considered healthy.

If we look at the previous four response abilities, they are in most cases, unconscious responses. The processes of perception, adaptation, recovery, and evolution are often automatic, subconscious processes that most people are unaware of. By making a conscious effort to improve our health and increase our awareness we become more perceptive to the subtle and sublime, becoming more aware of, and even participatory, in these four response abilities.

The fifth *response ability of expression* is a more conscious process by which we express physically, a mental intention. The simplest example of this would be to wiggle your finger. You create the desire in your mind to move your finger, you transform that desire into an intention, and then move your finger. Other examples are, to run from danger, eat food when hungry, and pursue your inner urge to find a mate.

After embarking on a clear path to healing, we may begin to experience the increased awareness of more subtle perceptions, and start to control and manifest previously unconscious activities that we now consciously recognize. As we learn, grow, and evolve through our life experience, we will act with conscious intention, rather than allowing ourselves to work unconsciously, on autopilot. An example of unconscious direction would be to allow ourselves to reach an extreme level of thirst, drinking water only when our primal instinct kicks in, acting like a wild beast who runs for the nearest stream. On the other hand, acting with conscious intention, we can drink eight glasses of water daily, whether we are thirsty or not.

In the same way, we could wait until we experience heart disease or diabetes before we give up hot dogs, french fries and cigarettes, or we can choose to eat more fruit and vegetables on a daily basis, preventing the crisis from occurring.

People have been known to slow their heart rate, control organ function, and adjust their own biochemistry through focused biofeedback and intense periods of meditation. This ability has a wide range of possibilities, but in order for us to achieve our optimum healing potential, this ability must be working at its optimum. For us to act in such a manner as to maintain our health and achieve higher levels of healing and wellness, we must be capable of acting physically upon a mental intention. When we don't, we exist merely as dreamers.

RESPONSE ABILITY #6

Harmonious Interaction

A bee enters a stream of wind and rides it across a beautiful field of flowers. As the gust of wind fades, the bee flies down towards the ground and lands on the petal of a beautiful daffodil. The bee walks across the petal to the center of the flower and sips its delicious nectar. As the bee drinks from this natural fountain, he rubs against the flower's stamen and pollen falls upon his back. As he takes his last sip, another breeze picks him up and carries him to another part of the field where he lands upon another daffodil. Once again he enters the flower to partake of the nectar, the pollen on his back falls upon the stigma of this flower, and a new life begins. This is pollination and it is the process by which plants reproduce.

We live in an interactive universe. Nothing works independently. The Earth is often called a "web of life" for all living things are inter-dependent. Without plants, bees would not have nectar to survive; without bees, plants could not reproduce; without plants, all animal life would perish because the atmosphere would lack oxygen. It is an endless cycle of interdependence.

In the jungles of South America, there lies a cave. Within this cave, lives two creatures – a unique species of worm and a unique species of bat. Nowhere else in the world will you find these two species except in this cave. What makes these two creatures so special is their unique relationship. Since the bat never leaves the cave and the only form of life is this worm, the worm is the only source of food for the bat. What is interesting, however, is that it is the excrement of the bat that provides the sustenance for the worm. The worm feeds the bat. The bat feeds the worm. The cycle goes on and on. This is called a *symbiosis*, two animals mutually benefiting from the existence of each other ... an example of *harmonious interaction*.

Healthy bodies, whether human, corporate, or the body of the universe, must be capable of interacting harmoniously with others. It is the harmonious interaction of the individual cells of our body that sustains life. Harmonious interaction of co-workers produce a thriving business and through the harmonious interaction of citizens a healthy society is found.

Through disharmony, separation, and alienation disease is experienced. Looking at our body, we see that all disease, especially cancerous, infectious, and autoimmune diseases, are caused by some form of disharmonious interaction between the cells of the body, or cells of the body and an outside agent. If relationships between all the cells of the body were harmonious, there would be no cancer or autoimmune disease. Conversely, if there was harmonious interaction between the body and the virus, bacteria, or other visiting entities within the body, there would be no infection.

Likewise of the world at large, you will find that all crimes, wars, and other social diseases are caused by disharmonious relationships.

When we begin to create more harmonious interactions within ourselves, accepting responsibility consciously, and allowing these interactions to spread into our relationships, we will find that harmony blankets the world with a sea of joy and all disease disappears. Once and for all, we would experience total health and enjoy the fullest appreciation of life and each other.

Only through this process of healing ourselves will we heal the world, and only by acting upon our deepest desires and intentions will we fully appreciate and develop to its fullest potential, the final and most important response ability – the ability of *contentment*.

RESPONSE ABILITY #7

Contentment

What makes the bee leave the flower? The nectar is so good and life-giving, why would it ever leave? Why do lions rest after the hunt, leaving a half-eaten carcass for the hyenas? Why do we balance our working life with vacation and play? The answer, *contentment*.

Studies have shown that mice will eat continuously until their stomachs rupture and they die if the hormone of satiation, or being full, is inhibited. Have you ever eaten a big meal on Thanksgiving? How did you feel afterwards, as you sat on the couch, your hands across your belly? Full? Yes. But also, content.

This feeling of contentment lets us know that a process is complete. Without this ability, one would never stop what they started, and exhaustion, eventually death, would result.

It is for this reason – to experience contentment – that we do anything. Contentment is present throughout nature and it drives life forward. Without this ability we wouldn't eat, drink, or do anything. Whether to survive, to procreate and continue our species, or to live to our fullest potential and make a dramatic difference in the lives of others, it is the resultant experience of contentment that pushes us to act upon our intentions.

Why would we take one step on this clear path to healing if it was not to savor a fuller experience of contentment? Whether your desire is to break free from pain and suffering or to experience your optimum health potential and a fuller expression of life, it is this longing for contentment that drives us.

Contentment sets the parameters of balance in our biochemistry. It causes our body to adapt to change and recover from the adaptation when the change is gone. It stimulates evolution and growth, motivates us to act physically upon our mental intention, and urges us to create harmonious relationships with others. This is the response ability that drives and completes the other six response abilities. The word contentment means "to hold together." The desire for contentment gives us the courage to take the first step, provides the persistence, confidence, and ardor to help us continue on the path, and rewards us with satisfaction and gratitude.

Now that we have examined what it means to be healthy, a new question emerges: Why do we get sick? What causes us to lose our ability to respond appropriately to changes in the environment. We will explore these questions and discover the answers in the next chapter – The Cause of All Disease.

1. "About WHO: Definition of Health," http://www.who.int/aboutwho/en/ definition.html
2. *Webster's Seventh New Collegiate Dictionary*, G.&C. Merrium Co., 1965, p. 383.
3. Guyton, Arthur C., M.D., *Textbook of Medical Physiology*, W. B. Saunders Company, Philadelphia, 1986, pp. 572-573.
4. Guyton, ibid., pp.923-936.

The Seven Attributes of Health : Summary

Health is the experience of being whole. Healing is the process of becoming whole. There are seven attributes – response abilities – that determine if something is healthy. They are:

1. **Perception** – Change is inevitable. We must be able to perceive this change.
2. **Adaptation** – We must be able to perceive this change so that we may adapt to it.
3. **Recovery** – Once the change is gone, we must recover from the experience.
4. **Evolution** – Change always leaves its mark, therefore, we must grow and evolve from the experience.
5. **Expression** – To act upon what we have learned, we must be able to express physically the intentions of our mind and emotions.
6. **Harmonious Interaction** – Since we live in an interdependent world, we influence others through our expression, and are influenced by others, therefore we must be capable of harmonious interaction.
7. **Contentment** – Through this whole process, we need to feel contentment to have a motivating force to drive us forward, and to know when the process is complete.

7

THE CAUSE OF ALL DISEASE

Thou sendest to man Thy messenger, the disease, which announces the approach of danger and bids him prepare to overcome them. ~ *Maimonedes*

When I ask the question, "What is the cause of all disease?" I usually receive one of two answers, *germs* or *stress*. Looking at our hectic American society, and all of its stress-related illnesses such as heart disease, cancer, obesity, hypertension, diabetes, and arthritis, it's easy to understand why people rationalize that stress is the cause. When we witness the association between bacteria, viruses, germs, and disease or illness, it comes to reason that they too, are a cause.

Every day our newspapers and medical research studies report that stress and germs are the cause of the majority of diseases in our world. Daily, we see countless advertisements on television and in the newspapers about medications that fight germs and relieve stress.

With all this "evidence" and the research that documents it, it would appear that stress and germs are in fact, the cause of all disease. Yet, as we learned in chapters 3 and 4, this is an illusion. Stress and germs are not the cause of all disease, but instead, the *cause of all health.*

Placing germs within the broader concept of stress, let's define *stress.* According to *Webster*, stress is a "physical, chemical, or emotional factor that causes bodily or mental change."[1] In other words, stress is any change in our outside environment that causes a change in our internal environment, whether it's of a physical, emotional, or chemical nature.

Example: Imagine you are walking down the street. As you step off a curb, you stumble and your foot twists under your leg. The particular way you twisted your leg, in relation to your current level of flexibility (or adaptability) of your leg, results in a strained tendon in your ankle. This is a physical stress. Did the stress cause the injury? No. It was your inability to adapt appropriately to that specific movement that caused the injury. If the tendon was more flexible (or adaptable) and you were able to respond appropriately, the action would not have caused an injury.

Other examples of physical stress can be a traumatic event such as a football injury, an automobile collision, or a ski accident. It may be something subtle such as carrying your purse on the same shoulder every day or sitting in front of a computer for hours on end.

Notice that all of these examples are of a negative nature, whereas the definition of stress makes no distinction of positive or negative. Other forms of physical stress might be a tickle or a hug; taking a warm bath or receiving a soothing massage. These are also changes in the outside environment that create changes on the inside.

Stresses are not always of a physical nature. There are also chemical and emotional stresses. Chemical stress can include food, water, smoke, toxins, vitamins, herbs, alcohol, sugar, medications, recreational drugs or germs. Some of these may be considered negative stresses, others, positive stresses.

Emotional stress might include divorce, hysterical comedy, bankruptcy, recognition, death, and marriage. Again, some may appear negative, some positive.

Everything we experience in the outside environment creates change in our inside environment. The effect these stresses have on our body and mind are not determined by the stress itself, but by our response to it.

Understanding this, does stress and germs cause disease? Of course not. The cause of disease is not stress, but our body and mind's inability to perceive, adapt, or recover appropriately in response to the stress. Does the streptococcus bacteria cause strep throat? No. Our immune system's inability to respond appropriately to the bacteria is the cause. If I took a strep culture from the throats of one-hundred individuals, all would have a positive finding, yet most, if not all, would not have the disease.

Does smoking cause lung cancer? No. The body's inability to respond appropriately to the smoke causes lung cancer, otherwise all smokers would contract lung cancer. Does stumbling off a curb cause a twisted ankle? No. The body and mind's inability to respond appropriately to the situation is the cause of the twisted ankle.

Let me again emphasize the cause of disease: It is our body's inability to respond appropriately to changes in our environment or stress. In other words, a loss of our body or mind's *response ability*. As you may have realized, this entire book is based on this principle. All health is the result of our body and mind's remarkable abilities – response abilities – to experience the outside environment and respond to it through personal expression. The more efficient and effective we are at this, the healthier we will be.

The next three chapters will reveal the seven responsibilities, or conscious actions, of the body, mind, and emotions. It is through these seven responsibilities that we learn to master the seven *response abilities*.

Before we do this, here's a story that illustrates all seven response abilities; how they may be compromised, how their loss can cause disease and how they heal. This story demonstrates the presence and the loss of the body and mind's response ability.

The "Mama Bear Incident"

One day I was in the forest. I walked along enjoying the beauty of nature around me. Lost in the serenity of the moment, I stumbled across a small opening in the woods where a mama bear was frolicking with her three cubs. She spotted me. She was not happy to see me. Rearing up on her hind legs, flashing her sharp fangs and pointy claws in my direction she gave a loud roar and began to run towards me.

Here is a wonderful example of *stress*. A sudden change in my outer environment occurs – an angry bear is running towards me. If I don't do something, a second major change in my outer environment would occur, I would become food for mama bear and her cubs. In order to ensure my survival, my body and mind – *my inner environment* – must express the response abilities of health, so that I may respond appropriately to this stress.

Step One: I perceived a sudden change in my external environment – I see and hear the bear. Step one is completed. *Step Two:* I must adapt to this change.

There are certain conscious and unconscious changes that must occur for me to retain my current level of health. On an unconscious level, several things happen: My adrenal glands begin pumping adrenaline into my bloodstream giving me a sudden burst of energy. My heartbeat begins to race and my blood pressure skyrockets, increasing the supply of oxygen and other nutrients to my muscles and vital organs. My digestive system turns off (possibly emptying in the process), remember, digestion takes a tremendous amount of energy, and at that moment I require energy for more immediate needs. My pupils dilate, getting bigger, so I can see more and see farther. I begin to sweat and my mind starts to race – that's where the one conscious decision comes in: Fight or Run Away?

I choose to run away. The bear takes chase. Quickly I climb up the nearest tree. The bear shakes the tree with her mighty paws, her teeth glaring in the sunlight. Unable to shake me loose, the mama bear soon loses interest and she and her cubs prance off into the sunset, leaving me trembling in the tree.

Step two is completed. My body and mind adapted to the stress I perceived, and I survived, retaining my current state of health.

For the purpose of demonstration, let's pretend that I did not pass the next step (recovery), that I don't recover from the adaptation to the stress once the bear goes away. Let's jump ahead twenty years into the future.

Imagine me sitting at home, forty pounds overweight, sitting on the couch eating nachos and drinking a cold beer. I am channel surfing with my eyes fixed on the television, my feet propped up on a table. Can you picture it? Sound familiar? Sound like someone you know?

My adrenals are still releasing tremendous amounts of adrenaline (anxiety), which I "treat" with valium at night, and a cup of coffee in the morning. My heart rate is high, and my blood pressure is through the roof (hypertension), for which my doctor prescribed a medication to keep under control. I wear glasses to correct my vision because, since the *mama bear incident*, as it is now called, I still tend to be farsighted (myopic). I have trouble eating heavy meals, because my digestion system has difficulty producing enough acid and enzymes to break it down (indigestion, irritable bowel, Crohn's disease). What happened? My body perceived a stress to which it appropriately adapted, but never recovered.

In this picture, my body is still responding to a stress that happened *twenty years ago*. My body and mind are still being chased by a bear, even though the incident is twenty years past, perhaps even forgotten. This is the cause of most disease.

The body/mind lost its adequate response ability, therefore each stressful experience adds to dis-ease and reduces its ability to respond appropriately to stress. Whatever illness, disease, or condition you may have, if you look back at your life honestly and with an open-mind, you will find a past physical, emotional, or chemical stress, or, an accumulation of such stresses, that you experienced and didn't effectively adapt to, or you adapted to and never fully recovered from.

If our body is an intelligent organism perfectly organized and orchestrated, why would it lose any of the seven response abilities, or its ability to recover? The answer, goes back to the concept of tone. As described in chapter 5, our current level of neurological tone, or nerve tension, determines how we perceive the world around us. Similar to the guitar string, one level of tension produces one note, and by changing the tension you can produce a multitude of notes on the same string. Just as a certain tension produces a certain note, a certain note possesses a certain tension. Therefore, every experience produces a certain neurological tone and every neurological tone produces a specific perception of that experience. Every situation we encounter, be it a traumatic event such as an automobile accident or a divorce; a pleasant event such as a musical concert or family picnic; or something as simple as biting an apple or sitting in a chair, every event produces a specific tone in your nervous system allowing you to perceive the "note" of that experience.

The nervous system has a remarkable ability to experience and respond to a wide spectrum of events and circumstances, each with its own degree and character of vibration and tone. Sometimes, however, the level of vibration produced by the event exceeds our nervous system's current level of adaptability. In other words, we have an "overload."

Have you ever experienced sitting watching television, while someone is using a blender in the kitchen, another person is drying their hair in the bathroom, someone is using an electric drill in the garage and somebody else is listening to the stereo in another room, when all of a sudden, you flick a light switch, and everything turns off and the room goes dark? What happened? There was an overload, and in order to protect the electrical system of your home, a fuse blew, breaking the circuit.

The nervous system has a similar protective mechanism. It is called a *Vertebral Subluxation*. A vertebral subluxation is a condition of the spinal cord in which the body changes the position and tension of the nerve tissue and its surrounding structures preventing an overload of stress that can damage the brain and other nerve structures.

The circuit breaker in the house is designed as a temporary measure to protect the integrity of the system. Once the surge of energy or vibration has passed, the circuit breaker switch can be returned to its proper position and the electricity is returned to normal. However, until this is done all energy stops flowing through the system.

In the human body, the majority of vertebral subluxations are self-corrected during sleep and through movement and breath during the day. However, sometimes the vertebral subluxation may interfere with the body's ability to self-correct, causing the body to become *stuck*, creating a "Catch-22" in which the subluxation and nerve interference becomes a self-perpetuating dilemma. When this occurs, the signals that travel through the nervous system, between brain and body, continue to be interfered with and the body can not function properly. The body *remains in the dark* and no energy can flow through it. There is an interference in the system. In fact, the word subluxation, when broken into its Latin roots means sub- "less than," -lux-, "light," and -ation, "a condition of." In other words, a vertebral subluxation is a *condition of less light in the body*. In this state, the body continues to function as if the stress that caused the subluxation is still happening. The body has adapted to the stress, but failed to recover. In chapter 11, you will learn about *Spinal Hygiene* and how to increase your nervous system's ability to handle greater degrees of stress and how to clear your spine of all old subluxations that you have been unable to self-correct.

This situation demonstrates that stress is not the cause of disease, but it is the cause of all Health. Stress causes our bones and muscles to grow. It causes our minds to expand and reach higher levels of intelligence and knowledge, and it gives us the wisdom and insight to carry us through life.

If we wish to build our muscles, what do we do? We exercise. Exercise places controlled stresses upon our muscles causing them to respond with increased growth and strength. The stress of gravity causes our bones to become hard and strong. Exposure to germs, such as bacteria and viruses, increases and builds our immune functions. If we wish to expand our mind, we place it under the stress of study. Think back to the most challenging time in your life. The breakup ... the illness ... one traumatic event. Isn't this the event that gave you the inner strength and wisdom to overcome challenge today?

What about the horrible rape that causes the woman to create a support center and help thousands of women to recover from similar situations, or the man who has the heart attack that causes him to make new decisions as to how to live his life – get a less stress-ful job, eat right and exercise.

When singer Olivia Newton-John found out she had cancer, it was a devastating moment in her life. Yet, as she moved through the process with faith and determination, and healed herself of this condition, she developed an inner power and strength that she never had. She now speaks before thousands of people, inspiring them with the message that the cancer was a blessing and her greatest gift, for it taught her the value of life and the power of the human spirit.[2] It is only through such stress and difficulty that we grow, evolve, and reach our optimum human potential.

Now, let us return to our story ... twenty years into the past.

I'm back in the tree shivering, watching mama bear and her cubs prance off into the distance. As I start climbing down the tree, let's look at a different scenario. Everything returns to normal. My nervous system was flexible enough to handle the amount of input – neurological tone – and does not go into *overload*. I recover beautifully and no subluxation is created. My pulse rate is calm and steady. My blood pressure and adrenal function return to normal resting levels. My pupils contract and my digestion turns back on. *Step three*: I have recovered.

I look around the vale in which I stumbled and notice scratch marks on the tree and a unique pile of feces on the trail that I had previously not seen. I observe a distinct smell in the air and see some paw prints and a few hairs scattered across the ground. I take careful note of all these things.

Let's jump again *twenty years into the future* ... instead of an overweight couch potato, the experience has driven me to become a fit naturalist, backpacking in the mountains of North Carolina. Walking down a path, I suddenly notice a strange smell in the air. It is vaguely familiar, but I can't place it. I continue on and notice a pile of fecal matter on the side of the trail. It too looks familiar, but could be from any number of creatures. Suddenly, I begin to notice some scratch marks on the tree, and I perceive an all too familiar change in the environment. I immediately and consciously, hold my breath, turn around, and very quietly, tip-toe away in the opposite direction.

Notice the difference between this event and my experience twenty years ago. I learned and evolved. I am now able to adapt to the same stress with far less energy and far less internal change, making the recovery much easier and effortless. The next time I will need only to notice the smell in the distance and I will adapt very easily to the situation. This is how we, as individuals and as a species, evolve and grow. *Step four*: I evolved.

This story is a metaphor to demonstrate the seven *response abilities*, the process of growth and evolution need not be so dramatic. The process that I am describing occurs in every cell and coordinates all biochemical and physiological changes in our body. If I eat a cherry, my digestive system perceives the change in its environment. It notices sugars, proteins, and other nutrients and minerals, and begins to adapt by secreting enzymes to digest the cherry. Once the cherry is digested, all the enzyme levels return to normal – it recovers. If I eat a new food I never experienced before, I will evolve. As you can see, this process occurs every moment of every day we are alive and it is this that sustains us and maintains our health.

As we learn, grow, and evolve, we begin to make more conscious choices and decisions. The whole perception, adaptation, recovery, and evolution process becomes consciously controlled. Rather than being a burst of unconscious organic, automatic, crisis-oriented, survival mechanisms, it becomes a conscious choice. We start to perceive changes in our external environment before they occur, and consciously adapt to the situations in a healthy, less traumatic way. By noticing the subtle signs of the bear, I was able to make more conscious decisions and pass *Step Five*. I was able to express physically a mental or emotional intention.

I saw the signs of which I had learned through experience, claw marks, bear smell, fecal material, hairs, etc., and mentally created an intention to prevent a similar trauma to that which I had experienced during the "mama bear incident." I perceived the change on a more subtle level, consciously adapted by deciding what I needed to do, intending my body to do it, and my body physically expressed the intention. What begins to happen when we utilize this fifth attribute of health – to express physically a mental or emotional intention – is we begin to orchestrate our own internal changes, participating in our own healing process. Rather than allowing random, external changes in our environment to create internal changes as crises, we take responsibility and take conscious action, growing and learning in the process.

Remember, the *Mama Bear incident* is merely an analogy or parable allowing you to understand the seven attributes of health and the process of healing. This process occurs every moment throughout our lives, in our cells, our families, and in our world. As we explore healing and the dimensions of health and dis-ease, you will see how these seven attributes intertwine everything, not only health, but relationships, family, career, finance, politics, government, and world affairs.

Our story continues ...

As I began to learn more and more about the ecology and environment of the bear, I began to approach the bear with the intention of further observation and perhaps future harmonious interaction. Observing the bears at first from a distance, following the same family of bears for many days over many miles, I travel with them, staying out of their line of sight, and smell. I don't want mama bear to perceive a change in her external environment that she must adapt to ... namely me, a possible danger to her cubs. As I continue to travel at a distance for a number of days, she begins to detect my scent. Since I am at a safe distance away, she smells me, but does not see me. I slowly move a little closer each day until one day she sees me. She is familiar with my scent but I am still far enough away that she does not perceive me as a threat.

I move closer and closer, building rapport with the creature, until one day we are standing in the same vale as twenty years ago, and she continues to frolic with her cubs. She watches me comfortably and does not attack. I am no longer a threat. She knows this because I took the time to build trust and familiarity. I am no longer a sudden change in the external environment that she must adapt to in an unconscious way in the manner of fight or flight. Earlier, when she attacked and chased me up the tree, she experienced the same internal changes as I had, increased blood pressure, dilated pupils, adrenaline rush, etc. She chose to fight ... I chose flight. Since that experience, she too, has undergone a process of learning and evolution so that she may now, adapt in a conscious manner, making a choice to continue playing. What have we created here together over time? We have created a harmonious interaction, the sixth attribute of health, and indirectly, the seventh attribute of health ... contentment. *Steps six and seven* – passed.

If this had been another human being, we would have communicated through words or writing, as I am doing here with you, and shared each others experience. Through our harmonious interaction you can learn and evolve without the need to experience the terror of being chased up the tree by a bear. You can learn through my experience, bypassing the unconscious experience of the first three steps. You can imagine the scratch marks and smell, without experiencing it yourself. If you are ever in the same situation, you will be able to create the necessary intention and tiptoe out of there just as I did, never having to experience such a traumatic adaptation from which to recover. This is what differs us from other animals. We have the ability to take conscious control over the first four response abilities – perception, adaptation, recovery and evolution.

This is the secret to maintaining health, inspiring healing, and achieving greater levels of evolution, growth, and life fulfillment, and this can be summed up in one word: *responsibility.*

RESPONSIBILITY

Responsibility is the key to all health, healing, evolution, growth, and fulfillment. It is the ability to perceive an external change in the environment *before it happens*, and then make a conscious choice to how your body and mind will respond. This is the meaning of a clear path to healing. Health need not be an effort. Healing need not be the result of disease and trauma. Health can be easy and effortless. Healing can be an everyday process of discovery, learning, and evolution. By taking conscious control of our lives, and accepting responsibility, we can begin developing our seven response abilities and begin to achieve what we all really want: A more joyful, peaceful, love-filled and freer experience of life; and a fuller expression of who we are and the unique gifts and talents we each have to offer the world.

1.   *Webster's Seventh New Collegiate Dictionary*, G.&C. Merrium Co., 1965.
2.   "Surviving Breast Cancer," *People*, October 26, 1998.

The Cause of All Disease : Summary

1. Stress is a change in our outside environment that creates a change in our internal environment.
2. Stress can be of a physical, emotional, or chemical nature.
3. There are no positive or negative stresses.
4. Stresses such as injuries, germs, and toxins, are not the cause of disease.
5. Our body's inability to appropriately respond to and recover from these stresses is the cause of all disease.
6. Stress is actually the cause of all health. Without stress there would be nothing to give us strength and cause us to grow.
7. Response Ability is our body and mind's ability to respond to and recover from stresses in our environment.
8. Responsibility is the key to health, healing, and growth. It is the ability to perceive an external change in the environment before it happens and then make a conscious choice to how your body and mind will respond in advance in a way that is in the best interest of yourself and others.

PART III

A CLEAR PATH TO HEALING

8

THINK AND GROW HEALTHY
The Seven Healing Powers of the Mind

Nothing is, unless our thinking makes it so.
~ William Shakespeare

In healing, as in any process, all things begin in thought. Anything we wish to create originates in the mind. Everything that currently exists in the world had its origin first as an idea. In building a house, the architect creates the image first in his mind and then artfully puts it on paper as a blueprint. In designing a new invention, the inventor is found sitting quietly over a piece of paper sketching a new idea. In developing a new scientific formula or theorem, the scientist is found in his lab, scribbling the equations or images on the chalkboard.

The creation of health, as in all creations, must first start in the mind. Once the mind is made up and the commitment and unwavering determination to heal has been made, healing is inevitable.

Where you are in your life right now is a result of your past thoughts, words, and actions. If you are unhappy with your current circumstances, and it is all you think about, then you will continue to recreate the same circumstances in your future. By creating a new vision of possibility, your future will begin to reflect that vision.

During my studies of human potential, I have found that there are seven powers of the mind. These powers, when consciously utilized, bring about the process of creation. *A Clear Path to Healing* discusses these mental powers in relation to healing and the creation of health; however, they may also be used to create financial abundance, loving relationships or anything else you desire in life.

Like muscle, these mental powers must be developed and strengthened through regular use and exercise. Throughout this chapter, you will be given exercises to begin their development. By using them regularly, you will learn to master them.

MENTAL POWER #1

Imagination and Creativity

The greatest mental faculty we possess is our ability to *creatively imagine* ... to create in our mind an idea or image that previously did not exist. Once this idea is planted in your mind, you then have the power to bring forth that image into reality.

It is important to realize that these images can be both positive and negative. You can create in your mind images of joy, health, and abundance, and you can create images of despair, sickness, and poverty. You choose the thoughts you think. You can allow pleasant or disturbing images to enter your mind. If I ask you to imagine your car, immediately an image of your car comes to mind, or if you don't want to see your car you could visualize your house. The choice is yours.

In regards to health, you must create the image of health in your mind that you wish to create in your life. When you are sick and feeling bad, it is common to think about illness. Remember it's your choice. Although it is more challenging to think of health and vitality when you are sick, it is necessary if you are to create the health that you desire. When you are sick in bed, you must picture yourself running through a field, full of vibrant energy with a huge smile on your face. If you want to loose weight, you should begin to imagine yourself exactly the way you wish to appear, healthier, more muscular, and full of vitality. As James Allen said in his book, *As A Man Thinketh*, "As we thinketh, so are we."[1]

Exercise 1

Write a detailed picture of the life you would like to create. If time, money, and ability were not an issue, what would you be doing? What would you have? What kind of a person would you be? Be exact. Make it your own. In this vision statement, address the following issues: Health, finances, career, family, home, contribution to society, spiritual experience, hobbies, travel, any other things you wish in your life.

MENTAL POWER #2

Intention and Decision

"And God said, 'Let there be Light,' and There was Light," is the famous phrase that set in motion the process of Creation as told in the Bible.[2] He did not *try* to create light. He intended there to be light and there was light. What does this tell us?

The initial stage of creating anything is *intention*. In fact, the English translation of the Hebrew can also be read as, "And God intended ... "[3] When you *intend* to do something and you have *decided* that you will and must do it, wheels of creation are set in motion. That which you have imagined and created in your mind begins to take form in your reality.

As soon as you have created in your mind the vision of health, prosperity, and all else that you want to create in your life, the next step is to intend to heal ... make the decision that you *will* heal. In making a decision, you have declared to the world that there is no other option. The power of *intention and decision* is the most powerful mental faculty we possess. Once you intend to do something with the absolute decision that you not only will, but must, there is nothing that can stop you.

Here is an illustration of the difference between trying to do something, and actually doing it. Try to pick up a pencil. Did you try to pick it up, or did you pick it up? You either do something or you don't, there is no try. It has been said that, "I'll try," is the coward's "no." In healing, as in all things, you either decide to do it or don't do it. As the wizened alien sage Yoda in the *Star Wars* movies taught Luke Skywalker, "Do ... or do not. There is no try."[4]

Once you have created the image of health and wellness in your mind, it is at that moment you intend to bring forth that image into reality with the decision that you will do whatever it takes, and you will never quit until your vision has manifested in your life.

Exercise 2

Create a statement of intention. In this statement decide that you will do whatever it takes to bring forth the image from *Exercise 1*, and that you will not quit until it has been realized. This decision will be the most powerful experience of your life. Make sure this statement is positive, personal, and in the present tense. Insert a date of completion by which you would like your vision made manifest. By putting it in writing, with a date, it creates a sense of urgency that accelerates the creation process.

Example: "It is my intention by June 15, 2000, to weigh 120 lbs. and live a healthy lifestyle by eating right, exercising daily, and meditating twice per day for twenty minutes. I will be vibrantly healthy and full of energy, and every day will be full of joy, peace and freedom."

Once you have created this statement of intention answer these four questions:

1. What twenty things will I gain if I *do not* make the decision to create this vision?
2. What twenty things will I lose if I *do* make the decision to create this vision?
3. What twenty things will I lose If I *do not* make the decision to create this vision?
4. What twenty things will I gain if I *do* make the decision to create this vision?[5]

By answering these four questions in writing, it will create the fuel to drive you forward to persistent action. If at anytime during your healing process you become discouraged, frustrated, or anxious, review your statement of intention and reread the answers to these four questions. By returning your focus to your vision, you create a powerful *Why* that will drive you towards your dream.

MENTAL POWER #3

Discrimination and Judgment

You have created an image of health and wellness in your mind and created the intention to fully experience this vision with the decision to persist and never give up until it has manifested in your life. Now, you must utilize your third mental faculty – your ability to *discriminate and judge.*

It has been taught by many that judgment is the deterrent of all good things. It has been said over and over again to "judge not," for in judging others you bring judgment upon yourself. When you use discrimination and judgment to suppress, or make wrong, yourself, your circumstances, or others, you interfere with your ability to live to your fullest potential and experience optimum health and well-being. One of the worst things you can do to your healing process is to begin judging things as wrong or bad.

However, when you use your powers of judgment and discrimination to distinguish between two qualities, and judge whether that quality is desirable or not for the realization of your vision, they are very powerful tools. Through your discriminating mind you can identify those thoughts, words, and actions that bring you closer to your vision, and those that draw you further away.

For example, as an individual I can distinguish between when I am feeling strong and vibrant, and when I am feeling fatigued and depressed. I can judge which of these two states I prefer. This is the mental faculty of which I speak. If you take one action that produces a desired result and another action that does not, you may judge these two actions, discriminate which is in your best interest (and the best interest of others), and then choose that action you wish to pursue again in the future.

When you have committed to your vision of health and wellness, you must then carefully distinguish between the thoughts, feelings, and actions that will help or hinder you from achieving it. You must nourish those that support health, and avoid those that suppress it.

Exercise 3
1. Write down ten thoughts that promote health and ten thoughts that disturb health.
2. Write down ten words that promote health and ten words that disturb health.
3. Write down ten actions that promote health and ten actions that disturb health.
4. Throughout your days, observe your thoughts, words, and actions and at the end of the day, journal those that brought you closer to your vision of health and those that moved you further away.

MENTAL POWER #4

Belief and Faith

In his book, *Think and Grow Rich*, Napoleon Hill wrote, "What you can conceive and believe, you can achieve."[6] Henry Ford said, "Whether you believe you can or you believe you can not, you are correct." It is now known, philosophically and scientifically, that whereas our environment does in fact influence our beliefs, our *beliefs* have an even more dramatic effect on our environment. Our perception of our environment *is* our environment. It has been said, "I'll believe it when I see it." But we know that you will see it when you believe it.[7]

In Wallace Wattle's book, *The Science of Getting Rich*, he explains the difference between one who uses the powers of the mind scientifically and one who is merely a dreamer living in fantasy. A dreamer uses the mental powers of imagination and visualization as described above. However, they sit daydreaming about their vision in their solitude, wishing and hoping that one day their "ship will come in." This is a step above sitting with no hopes at all, but in order for there to be the manifestation of the vision it requires two more ingredients: the steadfast purpose to bring forth the vision and an unwavering faith that you will.[8]

With unquestioning belief that you will be healthy, health will take place. No doubts. No question. No fear.

Let's go one step further. Rather than believe you will heal, *know* you will heal. From studying the seven principles of healing, we understand that thoughts begin creation and that every cause has a reproducible and duplicatible effect. Every cause will have the same effect, every time. If you do that cause you will get its effect. If you want an effect, you do the cause. The result is reproducible and duplicatible. Understanding this, there is no doubt that if you apply your mental faculties and utilize the seven responsibilities found in chapter 11, healing must result.

Exercise 4

1. Write down ten beliefs you have about health, healing, and the human body.
2. Using your mental faculty of judgment and discrimination, determine whether any of these beliefs may be inhibiting your healing process.
3. If there are any disempowering beliefs, change them so that they are empowering. (i.e., Change "It seems like I am always getting sick," to "My body seems to always be going through a healing process." Or change "There must be something wrong. My stomach hurts," to "My stomach is giving me a signal. What can I do to support it?"
4. Develop five empowering beliefs of faith regarding your body's ability to heal. (Use the beliefs introduced in chapter 4 as a guide, if necessary.)

Visualization and Affirmation

If you can see it in your mind, you can accomplish it. *If you can describe it, you can create it.* This fifth ability allows you to begin to make real, the vision you have imagined and to make concrete the decision you have intended.

When using this fifth mental power, you bring the details of your vision into the physical world. In your mind, you have etched in detailed the vision you want to create ... in this case, health and healing. You now begin attracting it into your world by creating it in your mind's eye through vivid imagery and visualization. Once this image is planted firmly in your mind, you then describe it in the spoken and written word. The two abilities to visualize and affirm, will begin to bring your vision into reality.

Take time each day, either in quiet solitude or during your daily activities, to visualize and positively affirm your vision of health aloud. Here's an example for the intention of weight-loss. "I weigh 130 pounds. I am in excellent physical condition." If this makes you feel as if you are lying to yourself, you can use an alternative affirmation such as, "I am approaching my ideal weight of 130 pounds. Everyday my physical condition is become healthier and more vibrant."

By *visualizing* your ideal image and *affirming* its existence as if it is already here or it is on its way, it starts to become your reality.

Exercise 5

1. Describe in writing, in detail, the ideal picture of health you would like to create.
2. Close your eyes and picture yourself as described in your ideal picture. Run the image of your vision in your mind in complete detail as if you were watching a movie of your new life in a theater. Watch it from the beginning to the end, seeing the ultimate outcome as well as the steps that took you there.
3. Write a statement of health, being specific, in the present tense – "I am," or "I am becoming,"– and positive – not "I am losing weight," but "I am slender." Below are some more examples to stimulate your creative imagination, but make sure to use your own. You are creating your vision and your world, therefore, create your own statements of affirmation:

- "I am living to my optimum health potential."
- "Everyday, in every way, I am getting healthier and happier."
- "My body is healing itself and patterns of disharmony are becoming harmonious and pure."

Here is a wonderful affirmation for prosperity:

"The wealth of the Universe is circulating in my life every day. This wealth flows to me in avalanches of abundance. All my needs, desires and goals are met instantaneously, for I am one with the Universe and the Universe is everything." (You may substitute "the Universe" with the word "God," if you choose.)[9]

4. Repeat your affirmations out loud at least ten times in the morning when you arise, ten times at noon, and ten times at night before you go to bed. Look yourself in the eyes in the mirror for the best results. To accelerate the process of manifestation, speak them with emotion and enthusiasm. Emotion is what sets energy in motion.
5. Repeat your affirmations quietly to yourself, with the vision in your mind's eye, throughout the day, and as you go to sleep. Replace the constant chatter and mental noise with the movie of your vision. Make your image of health persistent in your mind.
6. Affirm the new positive healing beliefs you created in the last exercise.
7. If a negative thought, picture or word enters your mind which is not in alignment with your vision, "erase" it immediately by saying "Erase!" or "Cancel!" and replace it with your affirmations and vision.

MENTAL POWER #6

Acceptance and Allowance

One of the greatest obstacles to healing is our resistance and our reluctance to let go. Our ability to *accept* things as they are in the present and to *allow* ourselves to move through whatever is necessary to heal, are the two most important things we can do. The power of *acceptance* and *allowance* are the most challenging mental faculties to employ, and the simplest to experience.

Imagine you are holding a piece of paper that describes your ownership of a piece of gold. This piece of gold is laying in front of you on the floor. If you are holding the paper with clenched fists, there is no way you can pick up and enjoy the gold. But, if you let go of the paper, you can pick up the gold and enjoy its beauty.

It's the same with our current belief system and model of the world and health. We hold on to our disempowering beliefs so firmly, that there is no room in our mind to allow for new empowering beliefs or for new levels of health to evolve. The reason is simple: FEAR. Specifically, the fear of the unknown. We are afraid to let go for fear that we will get hurt or lose something. By letting go of your current suppositions, you will experience a profound sense of freedom in which a new world awaits you.

Exercise 6

1. Write a statement of acknowledgment of your current health status. Example: "I have problems eating foods that contain dairy and sugar and I tend to be overweight," or "I have been diagnosed with a dis-ease that has been labeled as cancer."
2. Write a statement of acceptance of your current health status. Example: "I accept that I have trouble eating foods that contain dairy and sugar and I tend to be overweight." or "I accept that I have been diagnosed with a dis-ease condition that has been labeled as cancer."
3. Read your affirmation from *Exercise 5* out loud ten times and visualize it in your mind's eye.

MENTAL POWER #7

Gratitude

The surest way to begin manifesting your vision, whether it be of healing, riches, or anything else, is to have *an attitude of gratitude*. Be grateful for that which you already have, and be grateful for that which you want to create in your life *as if it already exists*.

We all know that it is easy enough to be grateful for something that is sitting in front of you, but to be grateful for something that is not yet there, with the faith and belief that it is on its way, is one of the most powerful things you can do. By doing this, you are creating the belief in your subconscious that the thing you want is already present. As this belief grows, your actions and outside environment begin to conform to your belief.

It is known that feelings of gratitude produce hormonal and chemical changes in the body that are healing, calming, and stress relieving. By living in a perpetual attitude of gratitude for that which you have, and for that which you wish to create, healing begins and the cycle of your mental faculties is complete. When you become grateful for the completion of your creative vision, it opens the space to create another, bringing forth even greater levels of healing, prosperity, and growth.

Exercise 7

1. Write a list of all the people, places, and things that you are grateful for in your life. Write at least 20 of each.
2. Write a statement of gratitude for that which you have acknowledged and accepted in the last exercise. Example: "I am grateful for the strength, healing and wisdom I will achieve from this disease condition that has been labeled as cancer."
3. Write a statement of gratitude for that which you want to create in your life as if it already exists. Example: "I am grateful that I am completely healthy and strong, and live a life filled with love, joy and freedom."

THE FINAL EXERCISE

Putting It All Together

In this exercise, you will create a final statement which will tie together all that you have learned. This statement once written, will be your vision and affirmation statement. Once written, allow yourself to change it regularly as you begin to experience new perceptions and further growth. The guidelines for this statement are:

1. Begin it with a completion or expectation date sometime in the future. Example: "It is January 1, 2001 ... "
2. Make it Personal. Example: "... and I am ... "
3. Add emotion and gratitude.
   Example: " ... happy, excited, and grateful ... "
4. Make it present tense. Example: "... now, that I am ... "
5. Write your vision. Be specific.
6. Write another gratitude statement.
   Example: "... and for this I am eternally grateful."
7. And finally, declare it so. Example: "And so it is."

MY VISION STATEMENT

"It is September 20, 2005 (my birthday), and I am eternally joyful, peaceful, and grateful for the life that I am living. I live each day with abundant health, joy, and vitality and I have a healthy and happy family who I love and adore, and who love and adore me. We have so much fun together and we grow together as a family every day. We are financially abundant. We can be, do, and have anything we want, when we want, and how we want. We live in a natural environment surrounded by forest. There are mountains in the distance and a flowing stream which carouses around our house into a magnificent lake. We have a beautiful vegetable garden and fruit orchard. Our home is of wood, glass, and brick and is beautiful and comfortable. We have a large back window which gives us a fabulous view of a valley, the stream, the lake, and the mountains beyond. The cows in the valley continuously graze happily and we see deer, raccoon, and other wildlife occasionally meander across the field. We have a beautiful, loving, golden retriever who provides continuous unconditional love and companionship to our family. In our home, we have an enormous library of classics, inspirational, motivational, and spiritual books. We also have a beautiful music room with a wide collection of ornate, exotic instruments from around the world. I am a respected, successful chiropractor, author, musician, and public speaker providing quality, loving care to all in my community. Anja (my wife) is a respected and honored success and motivational teacher. Having become a disciple of success, health, and love principles, our every desire, need, and goal manifests instantaneously for we are one with God and God is everything. For all this and more, I am eternally grateful. And so it is."

With these tools you have now created an image of a life of health, joy, and prosperity and your mental faculties are beginning to awaken. By using the exercises in this chapter on a daily bases, you will develop their power, and eventually master them.

1. Allen, James, *As A Man Thinketh*, Putnam, 1959.
2. Kaplan, Aryeh, *The Living Torah*, Moznaim Publishing, 1981, p.3.
3. Danby, H, Segal M. H., *A Concise English-Hebrew Dictionary*, Dvir Publishing, Tel Aviv, 1958, p.11.
4. Lucas, George, *The Empire Strikes Back*, Lucasfilm Productions, 1980.
5. Robbins, Anthony, *Awaken the Giant Within*, Fireside, New York, 1991, pp. 71-72.
6. Hill, Napoleon, *Think and Grow Rich*, Fawcett Crest, New York, 1937, p. 31.
7. Dyer, Wayne, *You'll See It When You Believe It*, Avon, 1990.
8. Wattles, Wallace, *The Science of Getting Rich*, 1902.
9. Robbins, Anthony, *Personal Power*, Audiocassettes, Guthy Renker Corp, 1992.

Think and Grow Healthy : Summary

In order for us to reach our optimum health potential and live to our fullest expression of life, we must apply the power of the mind. The physical world around us and the actions we take are merely reflections of the thoughts in our mind. Human beings have seven mental faculties, which if used consciously, allow the individual to create anything, including optimum health. The seven mental powers are:

1. **Imagination and Creativity** – You create new ideas and thoughts which do not and may never have existed. Create the vision of your ideal self using your imagination.
2. **Intention and Decision** – When you know what you want to create, create the intention and make the decision that you will and must make that vision a reality. Once you have intended to be, do, or have something with the absolute decision that not only you will, but you must, nothing can stop you.
3. **Discrimination and Judgment** – You have the power to judge whether something is desirable or not, in the creation of your vision. Through your discriminating mind, you can identify which thoughts, words, and actions bring you closer to your vision and which draw you further away.
4. **Belief and Faith** – Develop the unwavering belief and faith that not only you can achieve your dream, but you will. "Whether you believe you can, or you believe you can't, you are correct." ~ *Henry Ford*
5. **Visualization and Affirmation** – Create a visual picture in your mind and describe it in words. You can use visualization and affirmations to bring your vision into reality, programming your mind for success.
    If you can see it and describe it, you can be it, do it, and have it.
6. **Acceptance and Allowance** – The ultimate realization of your vision, depends upon your ability to accept things as they are, now, and allow yourself to move through whatever is necessary to heal and achieve your vision.
7. **Gratitude** – The surest way to manifest your vision, whether it be health, riches, or anything at all, is to be grateful for what you already have, as well as for that which you wish to create, in advance, as if it already exists.

9

HEALING THE EMOTIONS
Changing How You Feel About How You Feel

If there's ever gonna be healing,
there has to be remembering and feeling,
so that there can be forgiving,
there has to be knowledge and understanding. [1]
~ Sinead O'Connor

Healing is a process. It is a path that bestows great benefit merely by walking upon its soil. Often, we enter this process with the hope of reaching a certain destination, achieving a certain goal, or reaping a certain reward, only to discover that when we arrive, the path continues into the horizon offering greater rewards and larger goals. With this realization, we learn that healing is not about the outcome, but who we *become* in the process.

In chapter 8, we explored the powers of the mind and how you can use your inner faculties of thought and intention to create what you desire, including healing and health. You learned that it is your beliefs and world-view, that determine your reality and your current state of health. By learning to shift the way you think and plant seeds of a new vision, you begin to manifest your desires, experiencing what was once only a dream.

As you continue to journey on a clear path to healing, creating your vision and utilizing the tools presented in chapter 11, it is very common for different feelings and emotions to arise. Old guilt, anger and doubt may enter your mind and heart from out of nowhere. Likewise, new fear, anxiety and sadness may develop if you see no end to the path before you. Although all these feelings are shared by all of us on our healing path, when you are experiencing them yourself, you may feel that you are alone in the process. The world may suddenly seem like a very big place, and that you are the only one on the face of the Earth.

During the healing process, these feelings are normal. Every human being walks the same path and feels the same feelings. If you experience such feelings, know that you are not alone. Recognize these uncomfortable and frightening feelings for what they are – signs and signals that you are healing and that you are on the right track.

In walking the clear path to healing myself and assisting hundreds of people to do the same, I realized that there are seven emotions common to all of us, and seven *Processes of the Heart* that move us through each of these emotions. As you read this chapter, remember two things:

"The only way out is through," and "You have got to feel it, to heal it."

EMOTION #1

Doubt

I place *doubt* at the top of the list, because I feel that this is the greatest obstacle on a clear path to healing. When doubt is present, nothing is possible. We learned that what we think creates a vibration that attracts to it whatever was imaged by the thought. When experiencing doubt, we send out a vibration that states that what we wish to manifest in our life is not possible, therefore the impossibility is attracted into our life.

Doubt is like a tiny bead of black ink dropped into a glass of clear water. The water is forever tainted, forever clouded. If you focus on your vision, speak positive affirmations, and live in gratitude, you have no doubts. However, as soon as you allow the tiniest seed of doubt to enter your mind, your mind becomes tainted, clouding your vision and hindering the process of healing.

The doubt we experience may be directed towards our health practitioner or whatever procedure or protocol we may be utilizing. It may be directed towards the universal principles that govern the universe or towards the healing process itself. Whereas all doubt will slow down the healing process, the doubt that will bring the healing process to a complete stand still and very often send it into a tail spin, initiating a dis-ease process, is doubt in ourself.

When we doubt ourself, our talents, and our abilities, specifically, our ability to heal, it creates changes in our body both energetically and biochemically that make it impossible to heal and often cause our bodies to create dis-ease. In Candice Pert's book, *Molecules of Emotion*, she describes a study that was conducted to determine the effect of thought on our immune system. In this study, they asked for the assistance of people who had contracted AIDS. They divided the subjects into two groups. One group was instructed to look in the mirror each day and affirm positive statements such as, "I can heal myself. I am a wonderful, strong, and a powerful person. Everyday I am becoming healthier and healthier. My life is worth living!" The second group was also asked to look in the mirror, but instead to affirm negative statements, such as, "I am worthless. I could never possibly heal this disease that has no cure. Death is certain."

What they found is that in the first group, the T-Cell count rose steadily, whereas in the second group the T-Cell count plummeted and the subject's condition began to deteriorate. To confirm their findings, they then reversed the groups, having the first group do the negative affirmations and the second group affirm the positive.

Immediately the T-Cell counts started to shift, and the condition of the subjects reversed in both groups! Realizing the powerful effect of the experiment, they brought the study to an abrupt halt and had both groups begin positive affirmations. As you can imagine, as soon as they started declaring life-affirming statements, their T-Cell counts immediately began to rise and their condition dramatically improved.[2]

What this study shows us is when we experience the certainty and unwavering faith that we can achieve, all doubt is removed from our mind, everything becomes possible, including the healing of a seemingly "incurable" disease. As soon as doubt again enters the mind, the healing process is halted and our quality of life begins to deteriorate.

In his book, *Anatomy of an Illness*, Norman Cousins describes how he healed himself of an "incurable" disease called Ankylosing Spondylitis (A.S.). A.S. is a chronic inflammation of the spinal joints in which over time the spinal bones, or vertebrae, begin to fuse together. It is very painful and can often lead to organ dysfunction. According to the diagnosis, there is no cure, and the prognosis is death.

Mr. Cousins disagreed. He believed that although the disease had no "cure," the body and mind were capable of "healing" anything including A.S. So how did Mr. Cousins heal this incurable disease? He took very large doses of Vitamin C and watched funny movies all day. He proved that "laughter is the best medicine." Watching "Marx Brothers," "Three Stooges" and other early comedy teams, he caused himself to laugh all day. Over the course of a few years, Mr. Cousins treatment worked and he healed himself of A.S.

Had Mr. Cousins believed the doctor's prognosis and doubted his own ability to heal, he would have succumbed to the deadliness of this disease. Instead, he believed in himself and he healed.[3]

By becoming *aware – the first process of the heart –* that doubt inhibits healing, replace it with certainty and belief and accelerate the healing process.

EMOTION #2

Apathy

If you continue to live in doubt, and fail to reach the certainty and faith in your ability to heal yourself or in a healing facilitator who will help you, you may enter a period in which you feel *apathy*. In this state we no longer care whether we get better or worse. We may become lethargic and enter a state of hibernation in which we do nothing, say nothing and want nothing. What's the use? We're not going to get better anyway, so why even try? If doubt doesn't *taint the water*, apathy surely will.

In my healing practice, it has been my experience that at this point the condition of most people begins to deteriorate. I often offer a few words of encouragement and tell an inspirational story to lift them out of doubt, however, once they reached the point where they had given up and didn't care whether they got better or worse, there was generally nothing I could do to help them. It was up to them. If there is no desire or intention to heal, healing can not take place.

Should you be in a state of apathy, and have a desire to move on, the only way to replace it is with care. The only way to replace apathy with care is through *acknowledgment, the second process of the heart*. When you begin to acknowledge the wonderful healing power within you, all feelings of apathy fall away and you begin to participate more in your healing process, igniting a spark under the flame of health.

EMOTION #3

Anxiety

Quite often, we have complete certainty and faith that our body can and will heal itself, yet we begin to feel impatient in regards to *when*. We may have certain discomforts or symptoms that we understand serve an important purpose, yet they are very uncomfortable and inconvenient and we wish that they would serve their purpose already. This anticipation can often cause another emotion to arise in the form of *anxiety*. Anxiety is the experience of wanting something now, while understanding that it may not happen for quite some time.

Healing is a process and processes take time. Just as it takes time for dis-ease to develop, it takes time for healing to occur.

Comedian George Carlin eloquently said, "Time is something we made up so that everything doesn't happen at once."[4] And that is exactly right. The only place the future and the past exist is in our minds, specifically in our memories and imagination. The only time that truly exists at any moment is the present moment – now. Likewise, at any one time, we are nowhere ... that is, now – here.

Imagine you are in a boat floating on a river. As you career around the curves, flowing with the current downstream, you can only be at one place at any one time – exactly where you are. Where you have been represents the past, and the river before you represents the future, yet your boat can only exist here and now. When you leave that here and now, you find yourself in a new here and now, with the old here and now becoming a there and then. (Whew!)

Now imagine yourself floating in a hot air balloon. Soaring in the blue sky amongst the beautiful clouds, you look down to see the entire river from beginning to end. From this vantage point, you realize that there is no past, present or future. There is only one river. So it is with time. In our finite existence on the physical earth, we can only experience the *now* moment, just as we can only be one place on the river. Just as we can see the river in its entirety from above, when we increase our awareness and level of consciousness, we can begin to realize that there really is only one time and one place – here and now.

Another result of anxiety is worry. Worry is the anticipation of something terrible happening in the future. If you focus on your vision of health and stay focused in the here and now, like anxiety, all worry falls to the wayside. By placing your attention upon where you are at the present moment you can begin to *accept – the third process of the heart –* your current state and relieve yourself of anxiety and worry and begin to feel secure and calm.

EMOTION #4

Helplessness

If we never become aware of our ability to heal ourself and acknowledge the power we all possess, and continue to live in doubt and apathy, we will reach a point in life where we give up. In this state of mind, we begin to believe there is no hope and that our condition or situation that we are living in is permanent. We forget that everything is in a constant state of change and we lose sight of our bodies' innate intelligence and infinite healing capacity. We despair that all possibility of recovery and an improved quality of life is lost.

In this state of *helplessness*, healing is impossible, and unless we replace it with confidence, strength, and inner power, our condition may begin to deteriorate. When we begin to *appreciate – the fourth process of the heart –* the power of the healer within all of us and the gifts and strengths we all possess, the helplessness is replaced with power, and the healing process takes a quantum leap forward.

EMOTION #5

Sadness

When we experience pain, dis-ease, and other forms of suffering, it is difficult not to focus on the suffering. We know that in order to create health, we must focus on healing. When we want to be strong and vibrant, we must see ourselves as such. Yet, when we are constantly reminded of our dis-ease by our limitations and discomforts, it is a challenge to keep our mind focused on health. This challenge can often cause us to lose sight of our vision. With the overwhelming constant reminder of our condition, our thoughts may begin to focus on our suffering, our disease, and everything that we may be lacking. Unfortunately, by focusing on images of misery, it only creates more of the same – misery loves company. When all we see is our suffering, and we lose sight of our healing vision, what remains is *sadness*.

From sadness comes grief. Grief is the feeling we experience when we focus on what we have lost or are lacking. Again, by focusing on what we lack we only create more lack. Yes, I agree that a certain period of grieving is necessary in healing, especially when we have lost a loved one. However, when we can begin to focus on the joy we experienced with that person and the wonderful life they lived, the grief turns to joy and the spirit of their memory continues to live with us through the rest of our lives.

If you are feeling sadness or grief during your healing process, focus on what you wish to create and *affirm* it – *the fifth process of the heart* – everyday. By doing this, not only does your sadness turn to joy, but the image in your vision begins to manifest in your life.

EMOTION #6

Anger

When we overcome our helplessness, sadness or other emotions during our healing process, we may begin to feel *angry*. We may think, "Why did this happen to me?" We may have lived a life of virtue and responsibility and still entered some form of dis-ease process. When this occurs, we may feel angry that such a thing could happen.

In order to feel angry we must blame someone or something. We choose something outside of *ourselves* and make it the culprit. By blaming the culprit, we make ourselves the victim. As the victim, we become angry that the culprit has done something to interfere with our lives. In this state of anger, we no longer need to accept responsibility for what is happening, because it is their fault.

From anger comes guilt. Guilt is the experience of blaming ourselves for some past thought, word, or action we committed that resulted in our dis-ease. Even though long-term guilt can be very devastating to the healing process, it can actually be the first step towards accepting responsibility. By removing the fault from someone else and putting it on ourselves, it begins our liberation.

To free ourself of anger and guilt we must be open to forgive, specifically in the form of atonement or *at-one-ment* – *the sixth process of the heart*. When we realize that we are not separate from our dis-ease, we accept what is occurring and accept full responsibility for what has occurred, without the need to find blame or fault in another or within ourselves. True forgiveness occurs when we understand that what is happening is actually in our best interest for our fullest healing and we become one with the process.

EMOTION #7

Fear

I left this emotion for last because it encompasses all the others. In order for there to be doubt, helplessness, apathy, anxiety, sadness or anger, there must be some degree of *fear*. We experience fear when we are uncertain of our future and we envision in our mind only the worst. When we see no hope of recovery and no end to our suffering, we feel fear. When it seems that our end is near and nothing can help us, we experience fear. Fear is at the heart of all the other emotions discussed. As said in the book, *Dune*, by Frank Herbert, "Fear is the mind-killer."[5] By removing fear all together, we can eradicate all emotions that interfere with healing.

In its truest essence, fear is the absence of love. When we are in love, there are no limits to what we can accomplish. When we are in *awe – the seventh process of the heart* – nothing is impossible and healing becomes something that always amazes us, but never surprises us.

1.   O'Connor, Sinead, "Famine," *Universal Mother*, EMI/Chrysalis, 1994.
2.   Pert, Candice, Ph.D., *Molecules of Emotion*, Simon & Schuster, 1999
3.   Cousins, Norman, *Anatomy of an Illness*, Bantam Doubleday Dell, 1991.
4.   Carlin, George, *Carlin at Carnegie*, Image Entertainment, 1983.
5.   Herbert, Frank, *Dune*, Putnam Publishing, 1984.

Our deepest fear is not that we are inadequate.
Our deepest fear is that we are powerful beyond measure.
It is our light, not our darkness, that most frightens us.
We ask ourselves, Who am I to be ...
Brilliant, Gorgeous, Talented, and Fabulous?
Actually, Who are we not to be? You are a child of God.
Your playing small doesn't serve the world.
There's nothing enlightened about shrinking
So that other people feel insecure around you.
We were born to make manifest the glory of God that is within us.
It's not just in some of us; it's in everyone.
And as we let our own light shine,
We unconsciously give other people permission to do the same.
As we are liberated from our own fear,
Our presence automatically liberates others.

~ Nelson Mandela's inaugural speech
as written by Marianne Williamson

Healing the Emotions : Summary

There are seven emotions common to everyone which may arise during the healing process. These emotions are:

1. **Doubt** – When we experience doubt, we send out a vibration that states: "What we wish to manifest in our life is not possible," therefore the impossibility is attracted into our life.
2. **Apathy** – If we never become aware of our ability to heal ourself and acknowledge this power which we possess, and continue to live in doubt and helplessness, we may reach a point in life in which we give up. In this state, we no longer care whether we get better or worse. Healing can not take place in this state.
3. **Anxiety** – Often, we have complete certainty and faith that our body can and will heal itself, yet we feel impatient in regards to the *when*. Anxiety is the experience of wanting something *now*, even though it may not arise for quite some time.
4. **Helplessness** – In this state, we believe there is no hope and that our condition or situation is permanent. We feel despair and all possibility of recovery and an improved quality of life is lost.
5. **Sadness** – When we experience pain, dis-ease, and other forms of suffering, it is difficult not to focus on the suffering. When all we see is our suffering, and we lose sight of our healing vision, the only thing that remains is Sadness.
6. **Anger** – In order to feel angry, we must make someone or something at fault. By blaming them, we make ourselves the victim. As the victim, we become angry that the other has done something to interfere with our lives.
7. **Fear** – In order for there to be doubt, helplessness, apathy, anxiety, sadness or anger, there must be some degree of fear. We experience fear when we are uncertain of our future and we envision in our mind only the worst. In its truest essence, fear is the absence of love.

10

THE HEALING PROCESSES
OF THE HEART

There are only two ways to live your life.
One is as though nothing is a miracle.
The other is as though everything is a miracle.
~ Albert Einstein

As you continue your journey on a clear path to healing, emotions discussed in chapter 9 may arise and you may find yourself going off track. Even though the path lies clearly before you, you may lose your way, becoming confused, scared or angry. By focusing on your vision and doing the exercises provided in chapter 8, you will find your way back to the path, no matter how lost you may feel.

There may be times when you become frustrated or feel helpless and decide to give up, later to decide to recontinue your healing path. Each time you lose your way and find your way back, you will become more familiar with yourself and your environment, and those moments of confusion and upset will occur less and less.

On a clear path to healing, there are seven processes we all experience as we go through this losing of our way and finding our way back again. I have called these the *processes of the heart*, for it is through the healing of our emotions that we lose our way less and less and become stronger and closer to our optimum healing potential.

Whereas the *powers of the mind* are conscious experiences and require you to take initiative to reap the benefits, the *processes of the heart* are more automatic and a natural consequence of being on the healing path. You will experience them in the form of a sudden "A-Ha" or flash of inspiration that changes your perspective of yourself and your world forever. Most of these are unconscious, automatic experiences, however, you can use the *powers of the mind* from the chapter 9 and the seven *responsibilities for healing* in chapter 11 to accelerate their arrival.

Let's examine the *processes of the heart* and see how they transform our emotions of fear and doubt into experiences of love, joy and peace.

PROCESS OF THE HEART #1

Awareness

Why are you reading this book? Probably because you believe there is information herein that will aid you in your quest for healing and health. By acquiring knowledge you increase your *awareness*. When you are more aware of the nature of your surroundings, you are better prepared to make more effective decisions. By making these decisions, you experience a more successful and healthier life. By living a healthier life, you fulfill the greatest potential of who you are.

Awareness is the first *process of the heart* you will experience on a clear path to healing. As you practice the exercises that develop your mental faculties, and incorporate the healing tools in chapter 11, you will become more conscious or aware of the world around you, as well as the world within you.

The awareness may appear as a feeling of discomfort. It may come as a sensation of "something seems different." Sometimes it is a spark of insight or creativity. It may even arise as a sudden "A-Ha," in which you suddenly see the world in a new way. Awareness may come slowly, or in a flash. It may be painful or feel warm and comforting. However it appears before you, it will appear. By becoming more aware of the subtle changes in your inner and outer environment, and how your world functions, your ability to perceive change becomes sharper, allowing you a grander experience of the world around you.

This process of awareness is necessary for you to heal. The more aware you are, and the sharper your awareness, the more adaptable you will become. Those things that once caused you grief are now merely an itch. The strong winds that once knocked you down, become subtle breezes on your cheek. You will hear the lion from miles away, rather than waiting to feel its hot breath on the back of your neck. It is common in our society to wait till a problem becomes a crisis before taking action. When you become more aware of the subtle signals of your innate intelligence, you can begin to take action at the first sign of change and transform the possibility of disease and suffering into a certainty of vibrant health and learning.

With this new-found awareness, many of your doubts about yourself, the world, and the healing process begin to transform into certainty and knowing. That which was once held as disbelief, mistrust or skepticism rapidly changes form in your mind to a notion of understanding, knowing and common sense.

When you experience anything unpleasant such as pain, fear, anger, or sadness, the greatest thing you can become aware of is that these experiences are an aspect of healing and are necessary for your growth and evolution. Through these feelings you can connect with parts of yourself that may have become separate, alienated, shamed, or injured, regardless if they are of a physical, mental, emotional, or spiritual nature. You learned earlier that healing is the process of becoming whole. By becoming aware of these separated parts of yourself, you can begin to acknowledge them once again and invite them in to be a reunited part of the family.

Awareness Exercise

Let's take a walk. Take your book with you and go outside. As you walk, pay attention to how the clothes feels on your body. Feel the presence of your clothing against your skin. Experience the pressure of the ground against your feet with each step. Feel the temperature of the air. Is it warm or cool? If there is a wind, feel its gentle caress on your face. Become aware of everything you feel with your sense of touch.

Pick up a stone. Close your eyes and run your fingers over the surface. Squeeze it. Feel its hardness and texture. Rub it first gently and then firmly. Become one with the stone. Smile! Do the same with a leaf ... some soil ... and the grass. Rub your hands over the trunk of a tree and if you feel so inclined, hug it. Is there a neighborhood cat nearby? If so, go over and pet him. Feel the softness of its fur. If he rubs against you, feel his caress. Touch and feel as much as you can. Become aware of all the things available for you to touch.

When you are finished touching things, continue your walk. How does your body feel? Are there any areas of tension or discomfort? What areas feel good? What areas do you not feel at all? Scan your entire body from the top of your head, down across your face ... past your neck to your chest and back ... your arms ... hands ... abdomen and low back ... legs and feet. How do all these parts of you feel? Become aware of every part of your body.

What are you thinking? What thoughts are passing through that mind of yours? Are they happy or sad thoughts? Are they pictures, sounds, or words? Are you thinking of something you wish to achieve in the future or are worrying about something that happened in the past? Pay attention to your mind for a few moments and observe the thoughts as they enter and exit your mind. Don't try to change, correct, or fix anything. This exercise is merely to observe and become aware, not to change.

How are you feeling emotionally? Do you feel happy or sad? Calm or anxious? Angry or serene? Pay attention to how you feel emotionally. Are these new feelings or do you have these feelings often? As you walk, think about habitual emotions and thoughts you might have on a regular basis.

Once you are aware of everything that you are feeling (physically, emotionally, and mentally), breathe in through your nose. What do you smell? Notice all the different fragrances in the air. The grass. The flowers. Perhaps it recently rained. I love that smell.

Listen to the sounds around you. The wind blowing through the trees. The birds singing. A dog barking. Cars or bicycles going by. Take in all the sounds.

Finally, look around. Rather than looking at the familiar shapes that you are accustomed to seeing (trees, houses), look at the spaces between. For example, instead of looking at the leaves of the trees, look at the empty spaces between them. Look at the colors and the shapes things are made of. Search for new ways to look at familiar things.

Take in everything around you. The sights ... sounds ... smells ... sensations ... feelings ... and thoughts. These things make up the foundation of your awareness. By being present in the moment, and observing everything around and within you on a daily basis, your perception will become more sensitive and you will become more aware.

Sometimes when you become aware of something, the discomfort may increase. Have you ever had your arm fall asleep? You may have woken up in the middle of the night to feel a strange arm next to you. You throw on the light and realize that it's your arm. You rub it, squeeze it, and pinch it to get some feeling back. How does it feel when sensation begins to return to the arm? First it tingles, then it stings, then it burns, then it throbs, then it just outright hurts! After the pain subsides, your arm comes back to life.

When I started Chiropractic school, I was invited to a housewarming party of a fellow student named Helene. At her party, I met a woman named Cathy who was in a wheel chair. We began talking and she told me that she had been paralyzed from the waist down since the age of six after what seemed to be a minor fall. After the fall, the feeling in her legs began to disappear and after a few weeks she could no longer move them. It was now over 50 years later and she had never regained her ability to feel or move her legs. The party ended, I said my good-byes, after which I would sometimes think of her, but never thought I'd ever see her again.

Four years later, it was time for graduation. My friend, Helene, who had the original housewarming party, invited me to a graduation party. We were having a great time, when suddenly a woman walked into the room who looked familiar. I asked Helene who that was? She said it was Cathy. I couldn't believe it. Here was a woman who four years ago had been confined to a wheelchair for over 50 years, and now she was walking into the room!

I stared at her like a little child who was seeing an angel. She saw my stare, recognized me, and came over with a smile and said, "Nice legs, huh?" I laughed and tears came to my eyes. I asked her, "What happened?" She explained to me that she had been under Chiropractic care, for the last four years, getting her spine adjusted every day, sometimes three or four times per day. The process was slow, but the feeling and mobility had returned to her legs. I asked her what it was like, and do you know what she said?

"It was the most painful experience of my life."

This wonderful, true story demonstrates that healing can often be a very painful experience. Even though pain, discomfort, and other symptoms are increasing, it does not mean the problem is getting worse, it just means you are beginning to feel more. Healing is not about feeling better, it is about being able to better feel.

When you are aware of your power and acknowledge every aspect of yourself, healing occurs. You accept who you are, what you are going through, and who you can become.

PROCESS OF THE HEART #2

Acknowledgment

Once you are aware of an aspect of yourself that needs healing as well as what may have caused its separation or movement towards dis-ease, you can acknowledge that it is in a state of dis-ease, and your potential to heal it. The process of acknowledgment is a conscious decision, as well as an automatic response. *Acknowledgment* is the next step in healing and is necessary in order for you to move on.

Even though you are aware of something, does not necessarily mean you have acknowledged it. Very often, an individual may experience a healing process in the form of a chronic illness such as cancer, AIDS, or heart disease. They know that they are having this experience. They are aware. Yet, they may deny their experience in an effort to alleviate the pain and protect themselves emotionally. When we are told by our doctor that we have a disease or condition, especially those as socially cursed as cancer and AIDS, it can be very painful psychologically. We may think thoughts, as well as hear them from our loved ones, such as, "Oh my God. How can this be happening? What have I done to deserve this? This can't be happening!" By asking such questions, we deny that we are having the experience, and parts of ourself become separated from the whole. These parts of ourself that are suffering need our attention and acknowledgment in order that we may remember (re-member) them and unite them once again with the whole.

There is a joke that denial is not a river in Egypt. Actually denial may be a river in Egypt. Let's look at the story of Moses and the Hebrew slaves from the ancient scriptures.[1] This story from the "Book of Exodus" holds a profound truth about denial and the power of acknowledgment. You may have seen the movie *Ten Commandments* with Charlton Heston or the cartoon *The Prince of Egypt*. They tell the story about Moses and the Hebrew people being held as slaves in Egypt. This story is a wonderful metaphor for the healing process. The word Egypt in Hebrew is "Mitzraim," which translates to "from distresses or troubles."[2]

For four-hundred years, the Hebrew people were slaves to the Egyptians and their Pharaoh, and were forced to work under horrendous conditions. They were fed just enough to keep them alive. It was only when the Pharaoh's stepson, Moses, a Hebrew orphan, became aware of his Hebrew heritage that things began to change. Seeing the suffering amongst his people, he left Egypt, and wandered through the desert for forty years. During this time he became more and more aware of the importance of his people and his responsibility to free them. (The name Moses actually means "to draw out.")

After the forty years had past, he returned to Egypt to demand the Pharaoh free his people with the famous line, "Let my people go!" He expressed to the Pharaoh, as well as to his people, that the Hebrew slaves were the chosen people of the one and only God who created all things, and that He demanded that they be freed. Upon hearing Moses' demands, the Pharaoh increased the work of the slaves and decreased their food. The

Pharaoh was made aware, but this awareness actually caused the people to suffer even more.

Moses continued to make Pharaoh, and the slaves aware of their importance and the need for them to be free, yet the pain and suffering increased. The healing had begun. Ten plagues came down upon the Egyptians (symptoms?). Each plague came with every denial of Pharaoh, each one becoming worse and worse. After the last plague killed Pharaoh's son, he finally *acknowledged* who the slaves were and let Moses' people go. The people were freed and they experienced well-being for the first time in four hundred years. For once we acknowledge ourself and the awesome power we possess, we become impervious to outside influences. We increase our Response Ability.

The story does not end there however. Realizing what he had done, the Pharaoh once again denied the Hebrew people and followed after them, determined to destroy them. Unfortunately for Pharaoh, God had given Moses the power to split large bodies of water. Eventually the Hebrews escaped and the Pharaoh and his Egyptian soldiers drowned beneath the waters of the Red Sea. (*Interesting note: water was an ancient symbol for emotion.*)

The moral of this story: *Acknowledge* who you are and don't let doubt bring you down. By acknowledging the innate intelligence and the powerful healing abilities within you, you release the chains that hold you captive and you free yourself from the slavery of apathy.

PROCESS OF THE HEART #3

Acceptance

Becoming aware of a change within you or your environment, you acknowledge its presence as an aspect of yourself and an integral part of the healing process. You begin to let go of the anger, sadness, or fear you may be experiencing and accept the situation for what it is. If you do this with the attitude of "what is ... is," much of the anxiety and apprehension you feel will dissipate and be replaced with calm and security.

One of the greatest stories of the power of acceptance is the story of Victor Frankl, author of *Man's Search for Meaning* and a survivor of the Holocaust. Victor Frankl was a prisoner in the Auschwitz death camps during the Nazi occupation of World War II. Surrounded by the smell of burning bodies and the sounds of children's screams, Frankl found himself in an experience where death was certain.

One day, Frankl was taken to a dark room in the basement of a burnt-out building, so that the "doctors" could give him a "routine checkup." Before he knew it, he was strapped to a table and the men began sterilization surgery on him ... without anesthesia. As he lay on the table in excruciating agony, he had a realization. These men had the liberty to go where they pleased and do what they wished, but, they did not have the freedom to think for themselves. They were puppets of a dark master, of which they must perform such horrible acts upon another human being. Although they had liberty, he, Frankl, had the freedom to create in his mind whatever picture he desired and think his own thoughts. With this sudden insight, he accepted his situation and began spending all his time with his eyes closed imagining himself running through green fields with his children and grandchildren. He saw himself being free of his horrible surroundings and visioned himself traveling to America to share his story and newfound wisdom.[3]

Victor Frankl survived the death camps. He traveled to America and wrote his book, which has been a source of inspiration for millions of readers. If Frankl had not accepted his situation, he would have suffered through his experience and probably never survived. By accepting his appalling circumstance and creating a new vision within his mind, Victor Frankl not only lived through it, but healed himself in the process and helped millions of people around the world to accept their situation and heal as well.

PROCESS OF THE HEART #4

Appreciation

Your healing process accelerates when you reach the level of acceptance. At this level something magical occurs within you. It's as if you embrace whatever may be and welcome whatever may come. You understand and know that your body and mind are incredibly intelligent and wise, and that their every move has a purpose with your highest regard and best interest in mind. Even when things seem bleak and the process is uncomfortable and scary, you know that it is for the purpose of your healing and you can glimpse the light at the end of the tunnel, knowing that your vision will be realized at the end of the path.

This understanding allows you to *appreciate* everything – everything the body does, that comes to mind, and all that you feel. It won't matter how strange, uncomfortable, or frightening the things that arise may appear, you will appreciate them, for you know that they are in your best interest. Fear no longer exists and all doubt falls by the wayside. Your disease or condition is no longer seen as such, but instead is witnessed as a blessing in disguise. When you see the good in your hardship, you see the good in everything. Your mind fills with gratitude and joy, you are no longer prisoner to your condition.

This is the stage where victims become heroes. We have heard the stories of individuals who have overcome cancer by learning to accept it and appreciate its lessons. Olivia Newton-John – who tells us that if it was not for the illness, she would not have developed the strength and wisdom to pursue her life's mission and dearest dreams.

We hear of the man who experiences a cardiac arrest, acknowledges that he has been neglecting his family for work, and begins a life in which he makes his family top priority. He pursues a healthier lifestyle that incorporates a clean diet, exercise, and a stress-free job.

We hear of the alcoholic or drug addict who suffered their whole life with anger, self-hatred, and depression, suddenly admitting to their problem and discovering the inner peace and love that was there all along … who then goes out into the world to help others do the same.

These are all examples of the power of *appreciation*. When you begin to appreciate yourself and your world, you begin to care more about the person inside of you and the people around you. You release the deep-seated desire to participate more in your healing process and begin taking responsibility for your own health. As the helplessness fades away, you experience inner powers that come from within you, that have no boundaries or limits, and of which have an infinite abundance of supply.

With this appreciation, you accept your inner power to heal and manifest that which you desire. With each day that you experience this miracle of life within you and witness the changes as they happen, it's not something you have to think about. It becomes a deep, inner belief and you begin thinking about it and speaking about it the way you would say the sky is blue and water is wet. It is a knowing, and you begin expressing it through your actions and your words.

PROCESS OF THE HEART #5

Affirmation

At this point, the healing experience has become a very real and integral part of your life. No longer is it something that you desperately seek, nor is it a new idea in your consciousness. With everything that you have experienced, you realize that healing is an aspect of life that never stops, never leaves, and is your constant companion. Healing is not something that someone must do to you or the consequence of any specific action, therapy, or diet program. You don't require affirmations to remind you of its presence, and you don't need to visualize your healing vision. Your affirmations become your inner dialogue and the visualizations never leave your mind's eye.

You have read books, you have studied the words, you have followed the instructions. Healing becomes as familiar to you as breathing, eating, and sleeping. It is something that you do, just as your heart beats and your lungs breathe. You understand, through your own experiences and your daily increase of awareness, perception, and consciousness, that healing is not the relief of symptoms and remission of disease, but the constant process of growth, evolution, and learning. As your perception continues to be refined, and your ability to respond more appropriately, effectively, and efficiently to changes in your outer and inner environment, learning and growing become more a part of your regular daily experience. You begin to more effectively manifest physically your intentions, to interact more harmoniously with others, and experience greater levels of contentment, joy, and peace. Your disease, condition, or other expressions of disharmony that once caused so much distress, no longer hold a place in your consciousness and are seen as a consequence or effect of past causes (thoughts, words, and actions.) Your consciousness is filled with your vision and you witness the universal principles, that were once fictitious concepts in your daily life.

You emerge into the *process of the heart* called *affirmation*. Your encounter with every moment of every day reminds you of and affirms the truths, principles, and laws that govern the universe. You don't need to remind yourself of these things, for the universe begins to speak to you through life.

You'll notice your day-to-day language begin to change. You find that you no longer speak of lack or detriment, but instead spread only words of wisdom, healing, and truth. Affirmations flow from you as natural as your regional dialect and cultural slang. You are free from the prison of false beliefs, denial, and doubt. Your cup is always half-full, not half-empty.

Observe yourself in this constant state of affirmation and allow yourself to receive the voice of the universe through everything you see, everything you hear, and everyone you meet. Greet all experiences with open arms and realize that we are all one.

PROCESS OF THE HEART #6

At-one-ment

It has been said that forgiveness is the greatest healer. Whether we forgive ourselves for some past action or word, or we forgive another for something they may have done to us to cause us anger or grief, it has been said that the *process of forgiveness* allows one to let go of that which may have caused us hardship and move on to bigger and better things.

The process of forgiveness can be very healing and can create a new sense of peace and calm within, but it requires an inclination towards blame. In order for us to forgive, it requires that we first make something or someone the culprit of which we have been made a victim, whether that culprit be ourselves or another. In short, we are made a victim to the actions or words of another that has caused us grief. For a time we resent them, feeling anger, guilt, or sorrow. We may hold onto this event for years, until one day we no longer feel so angry or guilty and we let go, we forgive them. We offer them reprieve and as a good judge, we release them from their sin.

Although the process of forgiveness often can provide healing, it requires periods of emotion, belief, and mental activity that may interfere with health. The challenge of forgiveness itself often causes a great deal of stress and can sometimes create increased trouble in relationships. I do not disregard the value of forgiveness, however, I feel there is a process that accomplishes so much more, without the detriment to our well-being. This is the process of *atonement*, or *at-one-ment*.

Atonement or *At-One-Ment*, is the process by which you realize that we all experience challenges in life. We live each day with the same struggles and adversity that this physical existence offers. We have all been a child. We have all been through school. We all interact with others. We all experience joy. We all experience sorrow, pain and fear.

When you understand we are all the same, there is no need for forgiveness, because you realize that you are never the victim nor the culprit, and neither is anyone else. We are in this world together and we all have our ups and downs, high tides and low tides.

As we discussed earlier, people act based upon their thoughts and emotions. Where do these thoughts and emotions that create action come from? From our past experiences. Everything anyone does is based upon all they know. There are no wrong thoughts, words, or actions based on the person's model of the world. This is a very important concept to understand. Why did our parents act the way they did? Because their parents and other people in their environment had thoughts and feelings that caused them to act in certain ways. These actions influenced the thoughts and feelings of our parents, as children and young adults, creating beliefs and paradigms in their minds and hearts causing them to act towards us in whatever way that they did. Why does the criminal steal, the rapist rape, and the killer kill? Thoughts and Feelings. Thoughts and feelings created by some past experience. Maybe they were unloved by their parents. Maybe they were abused as children, physically or emotionally. Whatever it may be, something that they experienced created feelings and thoughts in their minds that allowed them to act in such a manner.

There are no victims. There are no culprits. There are only lost, hurt children crying for attention and asking for the love that they feel they never received.

You may ask, "What about children born drug dependent? Or genes that don't balance?" They still have the ability to choose. Many born into such life situations have lived great lives. One example is Tony Melendez. This man who was born with no arms, is one of the greatest classical guitarists alive – playing only with his feet! Christopher Burke, who played Corky Thatcher on the television show "Life Goes On" has a prospering acting career, in spite of his genetic disability of Down's Syndrome.

In 1882 a baby girl caught a fever that was so fierce she nearly died. She survived but the fever left its mark – she could no longer see or hear. Because she could not hear she also found it very difficult to speak. The fever cut her off from the outside world, depriving her of sight and sound. It was as if she had been thrown into a dark prison cell from which there could be no release. Luckily, this young girl was not someone who gave up easily. Soon she began to explore the world by using her other senses. She followed her mother wherever she went, hanging onto her skirts. She touched and smelled everything she came across and felt other people's hands to see what they were doing. She copied their actions and was soon able to do certain jobs herself, like milking the cows or kneading dough. She even learned to recognize people by feeling their faces or their clothes. She could also tell where she was in the garden by the smell of the different plants and the feel of the ground under her feet.

With the help of a teacher by the name of Anne Sullivan, she developed into an intelligent, young woman. She proved to be a remarkable scholar, graduating with honors from Radcliffe College in 1904. She had phenomenal powers of concentration and memory, as well as a dogged determination to succeed. While she was still at college she wrote *The Story of My Life*. This was an immediate success and earned her enough money to buy her own house.

This woman was very religious and her faith led her to examine the world more and more carefully. She began to realize that there was great injustice in the world and that people were not treated equally. Blindness was often caused by disease which was itself often caused by poverty. She became a suffragette and a socialist, demanding equal rights for women and better pay for working-class people. She also helped set up the American Foundation for the Blind in order to provide better services to people with impaired vision. She toured the country, giving lecture after lecture. Many books were written about her and several plays and films were made about her life. Eventually she became so famous that she was invited abroad and received many honors from foreign universities and monarchs. In 1932 she became a vice-president of the Royal National Institute for the Blind in the United Kingdom.

This woman who suffered her entire life with only the senses of taste, smell and touch is one of the greatest teachers, scholars and philosophers in American history. Her name – Helen Keller. *There are no victims*.[4]

When you begin to experience the world through the clear "eyes" of awareness, have acknowledged the inner hero within all of us, including yourself, have accepted the good and the bad, have begun to appreciate all that exists and live in constant affirmation of love, light, and healing, you realize at that moment that we are all the same and live in a perpetual state of one-ness. It is at this point that you have entered the sixth *process of the heart, at-one-ment*. As you live in at-one-ment, forgiveness is no longer necessary for there is nothing to forgive ... only love to give.

Living in at-one-ment, as with the other *processes of the heart*, is automatic and instantaneous. It is not something you do. It is something you are. As you move down your own path of healing, atonement is the natural consequence of becoming complete and whole within yourself. Your life is as your vision. Your heart is constantly filled with joy. Your mind is clear and true, and all you see as you look at the world and the people around you is gratitude, wonder, and a deep sense of awe.

PROCESS OF THE HEART #7

Awe

"I am so lucky to have been given this life to live, and this world to live in, and for this I am eternally grateful." What else is there to think, when you are living in *awe*. In *awe* of your world. In *awe* of others. And most important, in *awe* of yourself.

At this point in your healing process, there is nothing you can not be, do, or have. You are the creator of your own creation and of this you are in a constant state of wonder and respect. You may still experience occasional challenges, sickness, possibly fear, yet one thing never enters your experience again: suffering.

Through your own process of healing, growth, and evolution, you have come to learn and understand that all things are on purpose and everything is of your own creation, created from your thoughts, feelings, words, and actions.

In my practice, I utilize a gentle form of chiropractic care called Network Spinal Analysis. In this process, we use as little force and input necessary to elicit the greatest ease and healing response by the patient. Using this gentle approach, people have tremendous healing experiences. I have seen people rid themselves of not only pains and discomforts, but allergies, asthma, hypertension, attention deficit disorder, poor eyesight, poor hearing, depression, anxiety, even AIDS and cancer.

When people experience these tremendous changes in their level of health and quality of life, they often ask me, "How did I get such great results when you barely touched me?"

In turn, I ask them, "Are you surprised?"

They usually reply, "Yes. I am surprised. You barely touched me."

I tell them, "The power of healing is already in you. It only needs to be reminded. This does not require great force for it is already waiting to be released."

They usually respond, "That is amazing."

At this point, I will tell them, "I too, am always amazed ... but never surprised."

When you reach the *process of the heart* of *awe*, every moment of every day is lived with such an attitude. Everything you see, hear and touch around you fills you with wonder and amazement, yet you are never surprised at what you experience. Because of your awareness and understanding of how the universe operates and how you and everyone else is an integral part of it, your heart soars with glee.

At this stage, nothing is hidden from you. Everything can be accomplished and overcome. Your life is a continual process of healing, creating perpetual growth, learning, and evolution. You have walked a clear path to healing, and at this moment you finally recognize it for what it truly is ... clear, easy, effortless. And because of this, you look at the world in awe, just as I looked at Cathy, as she walk into the room, amazed – but never surprised.

In this chapter, and in chapter 9, you have explored the many experiences that are available to you on your clear path to healing. The most challenging, and the most rewarding, processes on this healing path are those of the heart. Your emotions and feelings guide your thoughts and influence your actions. When you understand them and allow yourself to feel them with complete freedom, you realize that it doesn't matter how you feel. It only matters *how you feel about how you feel*. That alone will determine whether you succeed in achieving your vision of health, or succumb to the strong influence of doubt, fear, and apathy.

You explored the mind and the power of your thoughts and beliefs. You entered your heart and examined how your feelings and emotions influence your healing process. In chapter 11, you will look at the body. You will learn the seven responsibilities we all have on a clear path to healing. You created your vision and acquired new, empowering beliefs allowing yourself to feel. You can now take action.

We have journeyed a long way together. Let's take one more step and complete the process. If you don't accept responsibility for your actions, and make choices and decisions that are not in alignment with your vision, your efforts are futile and health and healing will continue to be a struggle. However, by aligning your actions with your vision, health is a natural consequence and a certainty. Your experience of healing will be easy and effortless.

1.   Kaplan, Aryeh, *The Living Torah*, Moznaim Publishing, Brooklyn, New York, 1981, 258-498.
2.   Segal, M. H., *A Concise Hebrew-English Dictionary*, Dvir Publishing, Tel Aviv, 1958, p. 132.
3.   Frankl, Victor, *Man's Search for Meaning*, Simon & Schuster, 1959.
4.   Keller, Helen, *The Story of My Life*, Doubleday, 1991.

The Processes of The Heart Summary

There are seven *processes of the heart* which are natural consequences of the healing process. These seven process are:

1. **Awareness** – The more aware you are, and the sharper this awareness, the more adaptable you become and those things that caused you grief, are now merely an itch.
2. **Acknowledgment** – Acknowledgment allows you to recognize the awesome being that you are. By acknowledging every aspect of yourself, including the parts that cause you grief, you can then become whole.
3. **Acceptance** – By accepting any situation with an attitude of "what is … is," much of the anxiety and apprehension will dissipate and be replaced with peace and calm.
4. **Appreciation** – When you come to appreciate everything the body does, everything that comes to mind and everything you feel, no matter how strange, uncomfortable or frightening, your disease or condition is no longer seen as such, but witnessed as a blessing in disguise.
5. **Affirmation** – In this stage of healing, the universe begins to speak to you through life. You find that you no longer speak of lack or detriment, but instead spread words of wisdom, healing and truth. You free yourself from the prison of false beliefs, denial and doubt, and become one of the few who has a cup that is always half-full, not half-empty.
6. **Atonement** – Atonement or At-One-Ment is the process by which you realize that we all experience challenges in life. Each of us live each day with the same struggles and adversity that this physical existence offers. This eliminates the need for forgiveness, for in this state no one is the culprit … nor the victim.
7. **Awe** – When you are in Awe, everything you see, hear and touch around you fills you with wonder and amazement, yet you are never surprised at what you experience. Because of your awareness and understanding of how the universe operates and how you and everyone else is an integral part of it, your heart soars with glee.

11

THE SEVEN HEALING STEPS
The Seven Responsibilities

*First say to yourself what you would be
and then do what you have to do.* ~ *Epictetus*

In order to live ... act, In order to act ... make choices. ~ *Ayn Rand*

We have traveled far together on this clear path to healing. We have examined our beliefs and how they influence our experience of life and health. We have explored the universal principles which govern everything and applied them to understand the true meaning of health and healing.

We have learned how to use our mind to heal and create success in all areas of our life. We have seen how our emotions influence our healing and the *processes of the heart* we all experience as we transcend our limitations and reach our optimum health potential.

It is now time to take action. This need not be a struggle or an effort. Our actions should be an effortless expression of who we are. By first preparing our mind by creating a vision and deciding who we wish to be; the actions will come spontaneously as an expression of who we are.

In this chapter, you will learn the *seven responsibilities for healing*. After reading hundreds of books on nutrition, exercise, personal development, human potential, and spiritual scriptures and my own personal studies, I have found what I believe to be the core for a healthy lifestyle. The *seven responsibilities for healing* are:

- Positive mind cultivation
- Spinal hygiene
- Clean food and drink
- Complete breath
- Proper exercise
- Loving relationships
- Adequate rest

Before we begin, I would like to repeat one thing – Health is not something you must acquire. Healing is not something you must pursue. Health is the natural state of the human body when all interference is removed. Healing is the natural direction in which the body moves when everything is functioning optimally. Health should be easy and effortless.

The action steps that I teach are instinctual. If you watch animals, they do everything that I describe. However, humans have a strange need to make things more complex than they are. These action steps will provide you with the basic – the absolute minimum – requirements to sustain a healthy existence. You will find them to be easy and effortless to incorporate into your lifestyle. Let's begin.

RESPONSIBILITY #1

Positive Mind Cultivation

Although all of the seven steps on a clear path to healing are vitally important, without a positive mental attitude, you will lack strength and conviction to do what it takes to make healing happen. In the last three chapters, we discussed how to cultivate a healthy mind through the development and use of the seven mental faculties and the movement through the seven processes of the heart.

Begin this process by imagining in your mind the life and quality of health you wish to experience. Once vividly imagined, decide that you will create this healthy life and intend to do what is necessary to accomplish that. Judge your actions and thoughts and monitor them, discriminating whether they are moving you towards your vision or away from it. As you take action, have the belief and faith in yourself that you will create your vision. Continue to visualize in your mind's eye your vision and begin to affirm its reality through your communication. Accept where your life is at the moment and allow the new life of abundant health to manifest. As things change, be grateful for what you're achieving and receiving, and more important, be grateful *in advance*, for you have the faith that it is on its way.

Having begun to apply these *principles of the mind*, you can build a foundation of health from the core of your entire body – the spine and nervous system.

RESPONSIBILITY #2

A Clear and Healthy Nervous System • Spinal Hygiene

You have learned that to be healthy means the ability to perceive subtle changes inside your body and in the outside world; to adapt to these changes in an effective and efficient manner; to recover from these changes and return to a state of ease; to learn and grow from the experience, evolving to higher states of awareness and energy efficiency; to have an emotional or mental desire or intention and express it physically through your body; to have harmonious interactions within the cells of your body and out in the world amongst others; and to experience a feeling of satisfaction and contentment.

What do all these things have in common? They are all experienced, controlled, and co-ordinated by the nervous system. The nervous system is composed of the brain, spinal cord, and all the nerves. These nerves travel throughout the body connecting to every cell, muscle, organ and tissue, transmitting vital, life-giving energy and information from the brain to the body and from the body back to the brain. This highly complex system interconnects every part of the body creating a vast communication network in which every cell is harmoniously interactive with every other cell.

Because of the vital importance of the brain and spinal cord, the innate intelligence in creating the magnificent structure of the human body, encased these delicate organs in solid bone. Surrounded by the skull and the bones of the spine, or vertebrae, your brain and spinal cord are protected from any outside forces that may damage them.

Also surrounding your brain and spinal cord underneath the bone, is a durable membrane called the *dura mater*, or *meninges*, that provides further protection to the nerve tissues. Flowing between the nerve tissue and the meningeal tissue is a fluid called *cerebrospinal fluid*. This fluid flows up and down your spinal cord and throughout your brain providing them with vital nutrients, immune factors and shock absorption.[1]

In a healthy spine and nervous system, all the vertebra in the spine and the meningeal tissue move freely, allowing the cerebrospinal fluid to flow continuously throughout the nervous system. The meningeal tissue and nerves are free of tension and in a constant state of ease. In this state, the energy flows uninhibited, from the brain through the nerves to all the cells, organs and tissues of the body, providing all the information necessary to control and coordinate the body functions maintaining a continuous state of health and well-being.

When we experience physical, emotional, and chemical stress, or changes in the environment, the nervous system will change the tension and position of the meninges, vertebra, and other spinal structures to protect itself from an overload of stress energy. This change in tension and position is called a *vertebral subluxation* and inhibits the surge of energy from entering our nervous system, protecting it from any damage that it may have been caused. Unfortunately, this subluxation also interferes with the normal nerve flow between the brain and body which is necessary for optimum health and body function.

In most cases, especially during sleep, these subluxations are self-corrected by the body after the stressful situation has passed. However, because of its interfering capacity, the subluxation may interfere with the messages of self-correction, creating a "Catch-22" in which the body is unable to recover from this condition. When this happens, the nervous system remains in a state of adverse tension and malposition, not only interfering with normal body function, but also causing the body to continue to respond as if the stress that caused the subluxation is still happening (as discussed in chapter 7 in the *Mama Bear Incident*).

If this subluxation is not corrected, the resultant adverse tension and interference will cause the body to lose its ability to respond appropriately to other stresses and begin to lose its ability to perceive change, adapt appropriately, recover, grow and evolve, express mental intentions physically, interact harmoniously, and eventually its ability to experience contentment. This is the cause of all disease, including chronic illness, such as diabetes, hypertension and cancer; degenerative processes, such as arthritis and osteoporosis; infectious diseases, such as AIDS; autoimmune syndromes, such as chronic fatigue, fibromyalgia and irritable bowel; and emotional conditions, such as depression, anxiety and A.D.D.

Uncorrected subluxations have devastating effects on the human body and mind and are detrimental to your health and well-being. If a subluxation is present anywhere in your spine, it is impossible to reach your optimum health potential and the benefits of the remaining five health steps on this clear path to healing will elude you. If you are to get the full benefits of a healthy diet, proper exercise, complete breath, adequate rest and a loving heart, it is vital that your nervous system be free of adverse tension and interference in the form of subluxations.

The best method I know of to determine if chronic subluxations are present in your spine and to have them corrected if they are, is through the process of Chiropractic. Chiropractic is the philosophy, science, and art of detecting, analyzing, and correcting vertebral subluxations. It was discovered in 1895 in Davenport, Iowa by a very spiritual man and hands-on healer by the name of D.D. Palmer.

D.D. helped a deaf janitor by the name of Harvey Lillard get his hearing back by returning a malpositioned vertebra in his upper back to its proper position. The genius of D.D. was not that he discovered a cure for hearing or for developing chiropractic. The genius of D.D. was that he said that the human body has an innate intelligence that controls, coordinates, and heals all body parts and functions. That this intelligence functions through the nervous system and if the tension or position of the spine or nerve tissue is altered in any way due to physical, emotional, or chemical stress, that the body and mind would lose its ability to function properly. He named this condition *subluxation* and found that if the subluxation was corrected – as in the case of Harvey Lillard and the return of his hearing – the body and mind would once again return to optimum function.

Although the principles of Chiropractic have not changed in the last one-hundred-and-five years, being based on timeless universal principles, the practice of Chiropractic has changed quite a bit. Therefore, in choosing a chiropractor, there are a few factors that must be addressed and acknowledged. In selecting your chiropractor, there are a number of questions you should ask. The most important question you can ask a chiropractor is: *Do you correct vertebral subluxations with the intent to restore proper nerve flow?*

The reason it is so important to ask this question is that over the last one-hundred years many chiropractors have forgotten the principles of chiropractic and have begun to utilize chiropractic merely as another method to relieve low back pain, headaches, and other musculoskeletal symptoms. Succumbing to the demands of insurance companies and the pressure of the allopathic, medical model (refer to chapter 3), they have abandoned the principles of innate intelligence and healing to be accepted by the insurance and medical arenas. If you wish to get the full benefit of chiropractic care, it is imperative that you find a chiropractor who still abides by the universal principles upon which this wonderful healing art was founded.

Once you have found a *subluxation-based* chiropractor, it is important to determine what *adjusting technique* they utilize. Just as there are many tools and methods with which you paint a picture, there are many techniques available for chiropractors to analyze and adjust the spine. There is not only a philosophy behind chiropractic, and a science to support it, there is also an art to chiropractic.

In choosing your chiropractor, look for a practitioner who uses a technique which honors the body. There are many techniques that use high forces which can be adversarial and traumatic to the system. You want to find a technique that works with the body's innate self-correcting ability and uses the least amount of force to get the greatest result.

The technique that I have found to be the most effective, with the least negative impact on the body, is *Network Spinal Analysis*. It is a gentle, non-invasive technique using gentle touches on specific areas of the spine that reduce adverse tension from the meninges and corrects malpositioned vertebrae, correcting subluxations and returning the spine and nervous system to a state of *ease*. Through these gentle adjustments, the body learns to be more *self-correcting*. Acting more as a healing couch than a "fix-it" man, the Network Chiropractor assists the body to use breathing and movement to remove tension from the spine and nervous system and correct subluxations on its own.[3]

As you move through a series of levels of care, your spine and nervous system become more effective and efficient at dissipating tension and correcting subluxations. As the tension and interference dissipates from the spinal tissues, you become more aware of subtle changes in your inner and outer environment, allowing you to be more adaptable to stress and proactive in your healing process. (For more information about Chiropractic care, check out the resource section in the back of the book.)

When you achieve a spine and nervous system clear of tension and interference, the natural health and innate healing ability of your body and mind is restored, allowing you to be who you truly are – a creative, self-healing human being, growing physically, mentally, emotionally, spiritually, and socially.

RESPONSIBILITY #3

Clean Food and Drink

With your mind clear of negativity and your spine and nervous system clear of adverse tension and interference, begin focusing on what you put into your body. Everyday new books and opinions are presented which often contradict the widely held beliefs of nutrition according to the times. One day they tell you to eat low fat and the next day they tell you low fat causes cancer, eat fat. Then they tell you to reduce your protein and increase your carbohydrates, when the following week carbohydrates are bad, and you should increase your proteins.

Wouldn't it be nice if you could filter out the truth from all these opinions into an unchangeable system of eating and drinking. If you apply all the principles that you have learned in this book to what foods to eat and what to drink, there would be no question as to what you should put into your body.

Reading books on nutrition and fad diets from *The Zone* by Barry Sears, *The Atkin's Diet* by Dr. Robert Atkins to *Diet for a New America* by John Robbins, has allowed me to distill the commonalties and create principles of diet that are easy and effortless. These principles are in alignment with the seven principles of healing. They promote healing and they support health.

If you follow these principles of eating and drinking, you will never have to diet or change your eating program. Let's summarize these principles and then we'll go through each one in detail:

- Eat with a clear mind.
- Trust your innate intelligence. Listen to your cravings.
- Read labels.
- Don't ingest anything that doesn't sound, look, or smell like food.
- Eat at least 75% alkaline foods and 25% acid foods.
- Drink only filtered, purified, or distilled water
- Drink one-half your body weight each day in ounces of water.

By following these seven principles, not only will you get the nutrition and fuel you need, your body will begin to cleanse itself. Your body's innate healer will start to remove toxins, waste products, dead cells, and parasites. Your body will begin to build strength and stamina. Your ability to handle stress will increase. Your mind will be clearer and you will feel more joyous and calm. Are you ready?

I.   Eat with a clear mind.

II.   Trust your innate intelligence. Listen to your Cravings

It is important when you eat, to eat *consciously*. Often we eat on the go or eat so fast that we neglect to even taste our food. (I, too, am guilty of this.) When you eat in a state of hurry, or lack of focus, your body actually goes into a state of fight or flight, the opposite of digestion. When you eat on the go, your body is in a state of activity. Your body is prepared to confront challenge and take action. In this state, the digestive system goes into a state of hibernation. Activity and digestion are opposites. In this state, enzymes, acids, and hormones are not adequate for digestion and not only does your body not receive the nutrients from the food, but it can actually have detrimental effects on the stomach and intestines, resulting in such conditions as ulcers, irritable bowel syndrome, Crohn's disease, acid reflux, and many others.

When you eat, it is important that you sit down. Look at your food. Smell your food. And most importantly, taste your food. Take time, even if it's five or ten minutes, to really enjoy your food. Sit down, close your eyes, and clear your mind of stress and worry. Take a few more seconds to look at the colors and smell the fragrance of your food. By doing this, it stimulates your digestive system for digestion and nutrient assimilation. Put the food in your mouth, with gratitude for the food (for something gave its life for you to eat, even vegetables) and chew, tasting and feeling the food in your mouth. Close your eyes and experience the taste and texture. When you swallow, visualize the food becoming a part of you. See the energy and the molecules of the food becoming you.

You will find that it takes the same amount of time to eat this way. It just takes more attention and intention. After three days of eating this way, you will find a change in the way you feel and the way you digest food. Also, you begin to avoid those things that are considered junk and begin being attracted to those foods that are good for you.

All I am suggesting, is to enjoy your food. The questions of whether you should eat something or not suddenly becomes very simple to answer. You don't have to remember mathematical formulas. You don't have to carry charts and books with you for reference when you shop. You don't need to count calories, fat grams or percent protein/carbo's.

If you watch an animal, they innately know what to eat and what not to eat. If you put a human child in a room with an apple and a bunny, the child will eat the apple and play with the bunny. If instead you put a lion cub in the room with an apple and a bunny, the cub will eat the bunny and play with the apple. How did they know? They just know.

Within you is such a knowing. If you are able to clear the channels, first within your nervous system, and then within your digestive system, your body will know exactly what it needs and alert you to these needs through cravings. When our bodies are clogged with waste products and our nervous systems are interfered with because of adverse tension and past trauma, the signals become confused and our cravings become addictions. Addictions are merely confused cravings, that may be detrimental to our health.

By following the seven principles of eating and drinking, you can stop the process of toxicity and your will innately cleanse itself. You can begin trusting your cravings, for these are signals of your needs.

II. Read your labels.

III. Don't ingest anything that doesn't sound, look or smell like food.

These two principles are easy to understand and they simplify the entire decision making process of what and what not to eat. Read the labels and don't eat anything that doesn't sound like a food. For example, if you read the label and the label says oats, apples, and cinnamon, ask yourself, "Does that sound like food? Oats is a food, apples are food, and cinnamon is food. I can eat it!"

If however, you see partially hydrogenated vegetable oil, sodium nitrate, carrageenan, guar gum, blue #6, and high fructose corn syrup, you ask yourself the same question, "Do these sound like foods? Blue #6 and Sodium Nitrate definitely don't sound like food, and I am not so sure what partially hydrogenated means, so I'm not gonna eat this." See how simple this can be? For those times when you are not sure, use the following rule: "When in doubt, throw it out."

Why is this so important? If it is true that *we are what we eat*, it is important that we understand the effect many of these *non-foods* have on our body and mind.

One category of such non-foods are the *Excitotoxins*. Excitotoxins are MSG (Monosodium Glutamate) and *Aspartame* or *Nutrasweet* (found in most diet foods, artificial sweeteners and even toothpaste); as well as *hydrolyzed vegetable protein, texturized vegetable protein, vegetable protein, natural flavors*, and *spices* – all of which may contain from 12% to 40% MSG.

Designed as flavor-enhancers, these excitotoxins contain very dangerous carcinogens such as, formaldehyde (used to preserve the dead) and formic acid (the toxin found in ant bites), as well as powerful brain cell toxins (glutamate, asparatate, and cystic acid). These excitotoxins are known to cause severe damage to nerve cells in the retina of the eye with widespread damage to the neurons of the hypothalamus – the part of our brain which controls all organ functions, such as heart beat, breathing, and body temperature; as well as directing the hormonal command center of the body – the pituitary gland.[4]

Aspartame has recently been found to produce symptoms similar to multiple sclerosis and fibromyalgia, both muscular, auto-immune diseases. It has been found that when an individual experiences systemic muscle pains, it is very common that they use many diet foods and beverages which contain aspartame. They have had tremendous results once they removed these poisons from their lives.[5]

These excitotoxins are especially harmful to infants and developing children, for baby formulas and many of the processed foods children eat, such as breakfast cereals and fruit *drinks* are full of these dangerous toxins so that they taste *so good*.

Another category of non-foods are the bleached, fortified products such as white breads and white sugars. These natural and healthy products are actually bleached with the same compounds we use to whiten our laundry. This process is utilized to increase the esthetic quality of the foods, so they look pretty. Not only is the bleaching material known to be deadly to human cells, but it strips the food of all nutritional value. They therefore need to fortify the food with artificially produced vitamins and minerals which are barely usable by the human body. Whole grain breads and natural sugars, such as turbanado, fructose (fruit sugar), and sucanat are much healthier choices.

Since the cataloging of all non-foods is beyond the scope of this book, I can safely say that all ingredients you see which *do not sound like a food* are such *non-foods* and have equally dangerous and toxic effects on the body. Right now, go to your cupboards and refrigerator and throw out everything that contains such non-food ingredients. As you learn to identify non-foods you'll find your shopping cart will be filled with different things than you are used to. And you might find that you save money as well.

IV.   Eat at least 75% alkaline foods and 25% acid foods.

Of the seven principles of eating and drinking, this is probably the most difficult for people, yet it is the most rewarding. It is with this principle that you revolutionize what you put into your body.

There are many theories and arguments about what we as human beings should and shouldn't eat. Whereas it appears that our digestive systems were designed purely for the break down of vegetation, our bodies appear to require animal protein.

Explanation: Herbivores – plant and fruit eaters – have flat teeth for grinding, whereas all meat-eaters – carnivores – have sharp teeth for tearing and piercing. We have mostly flat teeth with a couple of sharp teeth (which appear to be flattening with time.) Herbivores have long intestinal tracts, whereas carnivores have short digestive tracts, we have long digestive tracts. Herbivores have a digestive enzyme called amylase to break down plant matter; carnivores have an enzyme called carnase which breaks down animal protein, we have amylase.

These are just a few examples of why humans are considered by some to be herbivores, yet there are other arguments in the carnivorous direction.

- Herbivores are able to stand and run within a few minutes to hours of birth, and are fairly independent immediately after birth. Carnivores, on the other hand, need to be nursed for weeks to months. They need to be protected by their parents, and they develop much slower than herbivores. Sounds likes a human child? Humans develop as carnivores.
- Carnivores tend to have long periods of time of activity followed by long periods of rest and inactivity. Herbivores, on the other hand, tend to be in a continuous state of activity, resting in spurts whenever they have the opportunity. Again, it would appear that humans behave as the carnivores.
- Herbivores tend to have their eyes on the sides of their heads, so as to be able to see what's coming from behind. Carnivores have eyes in the front of their head so they can hunt and see their prey.[6] Where are our eyes? In the front – carnivores.

As you can see, there are arguments for both. It appears that as humans, we have the qualities of both herbivores and carnivores. We have the need for plants and fruits, as well as animal proteins. However, what I discovered is a ratio for foods that is optimum for most people. This ratio will vary depending on the individual. Let's take a look.

All foods have one of two effects on the body, either an alkalizing or an acidic effect. Neither is good or bad, but most degenerative and chronic diseases exist when there is an acid condition in the body. If we determine a way to neutralize this acid and promote an alkaline environment in the body, many of our problems would disappear and our vision of vibrant health would manifest.

Keeping that in mind, it is important to remember that a food is either alkaline or acid, depending on its effect in the body. An easy way to remember is: all fruits and vegetables are alkaline ... everything else is acid. Therefore, meats – including chicken and fish – grains, nuts, seeds, sweets, and dairy are all acid foods. (Exceptions: pomegranates are acid fruits; millet and quinoa are alkaline grains; almonds are alkaline nuts; salmon may be an alkaline meat.)[7]

At least 75% of your entire dietary intake should be alkaline, allowing a maximum of 25% to be acid. Considering that the standard American diet is the exact opposite (75% acid and 25% alkaline) this can be challenging for some. A good way to change your diet, is to include one or two fruits with breakfast, a salad with lunch, and a salad and vegetables with dinner and a fruit snack between lunch and dinner. If you are one of the many who are eating 25% alkaline and 75% acid, work your way to 50/50, then 60/40, until you are eating 75% alkaline foods and 25% acid foods. (Vegetarians must also implement this ratio, for all grains, nuts, and seeds are acid.)[8]

Remember, the clear path to healing is designed to be easy and effortless. If you find yourself stressed over this, back up a little and make a slower transition. The intention and decision is to eventually eat 75% alkaline, 25% acid.

VI.   Drink only filtered, purified or distilled water
VII Drink your body weight each day in ounces of water.

One of the most neglected aspects of diet is adequate daily intake of clean water. One of the greatest contributors to chronic and degenerative disease, and the associated acid condition in the body, is *dehydration*, a deficiency of water in the body.

Eating a mostly alkaline diet will provide a wonderful supply of water to your body, however, it is important to remember that you take in a minimum, requirement of water everyday.

Before we discuss how much, let us discuss the type of water. It is important to avoid tap water. Tap water is full of chlorine, bacteria, viruses, and a multitude of toxic chemicals, metals, and carcinogens. Although, these things are not harmful in and of themselves (as discussed earlier), they do place added stress on the body, wasting vital healing energy. It is important to drink water that has been cleansed through a purification process, be it distilled, filtered, reverse osmosis, or bottled mineral water, avoid tap water and drink only purified water. Cooking water, the water you clean your vegetables and fruits with, and the water you shower with should also be purified. In our home, we have a filter on our shower-head that removes chlorine which might have otherwise been breathed in or absorbed through the skin.

The easiest way to accomplish this, and the least expensive over time, is to buy a reverse osmosis filtration system which filters the water as it enters the house. Through this system, every sink, shower and toilet produces clean, healthy water.

Another way, is to have five-gallon jugs delivered directly to your home. The cleanest water available is distilled. However, many of the trace minerals have been removed from the water, and water is one of our greatest sources of trace minerals. Therefore, if you opt to use distilled water, make sure to supplement it with a few drops of trace minerals which can be obtained in your local health food store or through the resource directory in the back of this book.

Knowing what type of water to drink, the next question is how much?

This is answered simply by looking at your body weight. Your body requires twice your body weight in ounces of water every day. For example, a 128lb. individual would require 64 ounces, which is equivalent to a half gallon or eight glasses, of water every day. Take your body weight in pounds, divide it in half, and that's how many ounces you need. For this individual, an 8 ounce cup (Dixie cup size) of water every 2 hours in a normal 16 hour day provides exactly the amount of water they need.[9]

RESPONSIBILITY #4

Full and Complete Breathing

Of all the nutrients and substances your body requires for optimum health, oxygen is the most important. Human beings are capable of going forty to sixty days without food and seven to ten days without water, however, a person can only withstand three to four minutes without oxygen before they die. If breathing is so important, why do we spend such little thought and such little time on breathing?

The breath is the gateway to your inner healer. Not only does breathing supply you with the vital nutrient oxygen, and expel carbon dioxide, it is also the main avenue by which you release tension and stress from your body. The body and mind release tension and stress in three ways: movement, emotion, and breath. If you do not express these three activities, your body will store tension in your muscles, tissues, organs, and mind.

We have all experienced the sudden surprise which causes us to gasp and hold our breath, as well as the final sigh of relief when it passes. This is an excellent example of how breath is an integral part of our experience.

Hold your breath for ten seconds. Afterwards, breathe fast and shallow high in your chest for another ten seconds. How do you feel when you breathe in this manner; calm or anxious; relaxed or uptight; healthy or sick? I think you know the answer. Now breathe in a slow, deep manner, down in your belly for thirty seconds. Now how do you feel? I suspect that at this moment you feel calm, relaxed, healthy, and peaceful.

Our breath is the metronome of the body. The depth and speed at which you breathe sets the tone for the rest of your body. If your breath is deep and full, creating a relaxed rhythm, the rest of your body moves towards ease. If your breath is short and shallow, creating a tightened, restricted rhythm, the rest of your body moves towards dis-ease. By focusing on your breathing, consciously intending to breathe deeper and fuller, your body will begin to move towards a state of ease ... a state of health.

Conscious Breath Exercise:

At least twice each day, when you wake up and before you go to bed, take ten full, complete breaths. A full, complete breath consists of the following:

1. Inhale filling your belly.
2. Continue the inhale, filling the solar plexus, the chest, until your head tilts back and your throat fills with air.
3. Hold for a few seconds.
4. Exhale, emptying the throat, bending the head forward empty the chest and empty the belly, pulling the belly in, emptying it entirely.
5. Repeat from step I.
6. A wonderful way to increase your breathing capacity and get a nice recharge of energy is to inhale, hold, and exhale in the following ratio: 1:4:2 For example, if you breathed in for a count of 4, hold for 16, and exhale for 8. A good exercise is to progress upwards as follows: 1:4:2, 2:8:4, 3:12:6, 4:16:8, and so on, up to 10:40:20 and beyond.

RESPONSIBILITY #5

Proper Exercise

All life grows through movement and challenge. The body and mind can only become stronger when given something that necessitates the need to become stronger. For example, when we wish to build our mind, we apply study, when we wish to build our muscles, we apply weights. "If we don't use it, we lose it."

This is what distinguishes a living thing from a non-living thing. A broom stick wears with use and is preserved through not being used. A living thing, in the form of a muscle, organ, cell, or mind, wears when it is not used or misused, and is strengthened with regular use. This is why we exercise.

In past generations, regular, disciplined exercise was unnecessary, for daily routines provided adequate movement and challenge for our bodies. Physical labor was more strenuous and more common than it is today. Most people hunted and gathered, farmed, worked in factories, and in specialty merchandising in the form of blacksmithing, carpentry, animal husbandry, and other such manual labors.

Today, with the advent of mass production, robotics, computers, and technology, the level of manual labor is greatly reduced, and often eliminated. Because of our sedentary lifestyles, sitting at desks in front of computers for hours each day, driving in cars for hours at a stretch, we must create the time to include the necessary activity for life and health to maintain itself: exercise.

The Exercise Exercise:

While there are many things we can do to exercise our bodies, there is the one bare necessity that we all need. When maintained daily, it prevents the body from wear and provides the movement and challenge necessary to create strong bones, muscles and organs. It is *walking*.

In order to get minimum exercise, walk 20 minutes 3-5 times per week. As you you walk, take long strides, swing your arms, and take long, deep breaths as outlined in step four.

If you find walking too simple, you can swim, run, play sports, work out in a gym, do aerobics, Tai Chi, Yoga, and hundreds of others activities that are available. As long as you do 20 minutes of challenging activity three to five times per week, you will achieve the bare minimum of exercise needed to reduce the risk of degenerative disease, reverse existing health challenges, and promote strength and vitality.

RESPONSIBILITY #6

Loving Relationships

Through *Love* all things are accomplished, for it is through Love that all things grow. It is the loving warmth of the Sun and nurturing bath of water that allows a plant to eventually flower and fruit. Only through a mother's love can a baby grow to be a child and eventually a loving person. It is through love that a lion becomes a kitten, and a bear a puppy. *Through Love all things are created*, including our universe.

The basis of spirituality is Love. "Do unto others as you would have them do unto you." Treat another being as you would want another to treat you. In a world created by Love, one can only be Love. As an apple seed produces an apple tree, and the orange seed only the orange – only can the seed of love produce the fruit of love.

"Act locally, think globally." Every action you take, every thought you think, has the power to change the world – and it does. The Butterfly effect states that the slightest movement of air created by the movement of a butterfly wing in the fields of Kansas, has the potential to cause a chain of events in the atmosphere to eventually create a typhoon off the coast of Indonesia.[10] This theory presents the idea that a small action can create a large result. In healing, often the less we do the more powerful the result. The world-changing, powerful work of Gandhi was performed by sitting quiet and being love. In the world of medicine, they have found that "Kinesthetic Tactile Stimulation Therapy" (Hugging, rubbing, and touching the patients) produces quicker recovery.[11] Only through love is there healing.

A recent medical study on the effects of cholesterol on cardiovascular health revealed a startling finding about the healing power of love. The researchers injected cholesterol into the blood of rabbits, and then killed them (not a very loving gesture) to examine them for signs of arteriosclerosis, or hardening of the arteries. There were two groups in this study, the control group who received no cholesterol and the test group that received the cholesterol.

The control group, of course, showed no sign of arteriosclerosis. The test group, however, revealed very peculiar findings. Whereas all the rabbits in this group received the same level of cholesterol, one half of the rabbits in this group had arteriosclerosis and the other did not. The scientists were baffled. Their conclusion was that whoever was responsible for administering the cholesterol to the rabbits forgot or failed to give half the rabbits the proper dosage ... until they met the little lady and discovered the real reason.

It turns out that the giver of cholesterol was a very little lady. The rabbits' cages were stacked up to the ceiling. She gave the cholesterol to the rabbits in the higher cages, that she could not reach, with a long stick. The rabbits in the lower cages, however, she would take out, call them by names, pet them, stroke them, kiss them, love them, before giving them the cholesterol. It turned out that the rabbits in the test group who did not have arteriosclerosis were the same rabbits that were given the love and affection.

To verify these findings, they repeated the experiment with three groups: a group without cholesterol, a group with cholesterol, and a group with cholesterol and love. The findings were the same. Those that received cholesterol showed the presence of arteriosclerosis, whereas those that did not receive cholesterol, and the group that received cholesterol and love, both did not show any sign of arteriosclerosis anywhere in their bodies. This study scientifically demonstrated the healing power of love. [12, 13]

If you are driving down the road and in front of you is a car with the blinker on, wishing to come into your lane, and you speed up with animosity to prevent them from entering, the effect of this behavior can be devastating for that person (unless they are living in love). This action can anger them, making them act angrily to their employee, and that employee in turn acts angrily to the cashier at the local market, who acts angrily to the next customer, who goes home and angrily beats his wife and child ... who never grows up to be the leader he was destined to be out of fear of being rejected and abused by others.

However, if you smiled and happily let that driver into the lane in front of you with love, that act of kindness would spread the healing power of love greater and faster than the wave of anger had, producing an endless chain reaction of love and kindness throughout our communities, our country, and the entire world.

Love is the answer to all the world's problems. It is the cure for all disease, war, crime, and hardship. It is lack of love that drives a child to become the drug addict or criminal. Most mental and emotional difficulties stem from childhood abuse or neglect – an experience of lovelessness from the ones whom we need the greatest love – from our mother and father.

We are born with the ability to love fully and purely. It is only through lack of love and fear that we lose this ability. For fear is the absence of love, as darkness is the absence of light and death, the absence of life.

It is said that we must forgive all, especially ourselves. As stated earlier, there is no truth in this, for in order to forgive someone we must first blame them – make them the scoundrel, the criminal, the bad one. We must judge in order to forgive.

Instead, we must remember them for who they are with compassion, wisdom and understanding – a spiritual being, having a physical experience with the same life challenges as us. It is only because of past lovelessness that they acquired the naiveté and fear or anger that caused them to act this way. If we act upon them with love, understanding, and compassion, there is no need for forgiveness. Forgiving is for-giving. Those who we are told to forgive, we must simply give love and understanding. They know not what they do.

It is with this understanding, that you move forward into a bigger, better world. A world of Heaven on Earth. At any moment in time, there is only one question ... What would love do now?

Throughout life, we are taught by our parents, teachers, doctors, and especially by television advertisements, that if we experience any form of symptom, ailment, or dis-ease, that we are sick, and we must stop these symptoms at all costs.

What they have neglected to tell us is that all symptoms are natural and intelligent functions of the body to heal. All symptoms serve a very important function. Regardless of where or how they occur, all symptoms and dis-ease are signs that your physical, emotional, or spiritual self is in a state of change or in dire need of change. When you experience symptoms, you are not sick, you are needy.

To shut down these natural healing functions with medication or therapies is akin to gagging a crying child's mouth. When a child is in distress and crying, we do not turn him or her away. We approach them with love and ask them what the problem is and what we can do to help. This is the same approach you must take in your own healing process. You must form this love and trust relationship within yourself.

From now on, when you experience any sort of discomfort, instead of running to the medicine cabinet to numb yourself of the experience and "gag the child," try to communicate with that area of the body. Console yourself internally, saying in your mind, "I understand that you are having difficulty and it is okay. I am here for you now. What can I do to help?" Take a few deep breaths, gently touch or rub the "crying" part, sending loving thoughts and understanding to the distressed area, just as you would for an injured child.

Children are very aware of this. Have you ever watched a child after they have fallen and scratched their knee? They wrap their arms around their legs, rub the "hurt" area, rock their bodies back and forth, and they moan. It may look pathetic, however, five minutes later, they are back playing again, their bleeding knee forgotten.

This simple change in perspective can dramatically change your healing experience. Next time you find yourself saying such things as, "My ... is killing me," or "This is my bad ...," change your perspective to "What in my lifestyle is killing my ..., creating a need for this change (symptom), and what can I do to support it?"

With this one small change in the way you think about illness, you will feel the innate healing power within, begin to change it.

RESPONSIBILITY #7

Adequate Rest

Finally, when you have finished your journey, *you must rest.* There are many types of rest and on this path I discuss four: Sleep, Meditation, Prayer and Thanksgiving.

Sleep – Your Silent Time of Healing

We are all familiar with sleep. We do it every night. Yet, many people do not fully understand the value of sleep or get the full amount of sleep that they require. Did you know that over 50% of Americans suffer from sleep disorders?[14] This is very dramatic when you understand the importance it has in our lives.

It is during sleep that the greatest and most significant healing takes place. During this silent time of physical and mental inactivity your body performs the majority of digestion, toxin elimination, self-repair and growth. Mentally, it is during this time that your mind and nervous system catalogue and integrate into your psyche, all the events and information experienced throughout the day, allowing for increased mental acuity, cognitive ability, expanded awareness, and continual development of the seven mental faculties. Only when you receive sufficient sleep do you acquire the benefits thereof.

When you do not get enough sleep, or a poor quality sleep, your body and mind are unable to integrate anything new, grow from experience, or become more whole in the process of healing. Whatever you can do to improve the quality of your sleep will improve the quality of your health on all levels.

Here are a few suggestions for improving the quality of your sleep:

I.   Maintain spinal posture while sleeping

Sleep either on your side or your back, supporting your neck and low back. Avoid sleeping on your stomach causing the neck to rotate. Make sure your knees are bent, putting a pillow under the knees if on your back. Whether you are on your back or side, make sure your pillow is the proper size for you, keeping the head in a neutral position, not bent forward or to the sides.

II.   Make sure the room is well-ventilated with fresh air.

Using an overhead ceiling fan and keeping a window open is a wonderful way to keep the room well-ventilated, providing adequate fresh air and oxygen during your sleeping hours.

III.   Use Magnetic and Far-Infrared Sleep Systems

Our earth is a large magnet. In order for life to exist on this planet, magnetism must be present. Due to steel and concrete, as well as electromagnetic pollution from wires, appliances, and cellular phones, the magnetic field of the Earth is depleted. It is common to feel drained and somewhat ill when in an office for many hours, and to feel refreshed and vitalized once you step outside. By sleeping on a magnetic sleep system, it provides a magnetic nutrient while you sleep, assisting your body in the regenerating, detoxification, and healing process. Many people have claimed an increased level of health and vitality after sleeping on a magnetic sleep system, even though they require one-quarter to three-quarters the amount of sleep they previously required without the sleep system.

Another technology that is available is Far-Infrared. Many magnetic sleep systems incorporate Far-Infrared technologies in the form of pillows and quilts. Far-Infrared energy is both the beneficial warming energy from the Sun and the warmth that radiates from our bodies. When you sleep under a far-infrared quilt, it regulates your body's temperature based upon your body's needs. If your body is hot, the quilt will draw the excess heat energy into itself and dissipate it into the atmosphere. If you are cold and require warmth, it will both reflect your body's heat back into you and absorb heat energy from the atmosphere and reflect into your body. Often two people can sleep under the same quilt, where one is cold and is warmed and the other is hot and is cooled. Far-Infrared technologies are also being used in clothing, especially socks and underwear, support wraps for the joints, and in some parts of the world, in carpeting and wallpaper.

These two technologies, Magnetics and Far-Infrared are a wonderful adjunct to your normal sleep products creating a sleep system that helps you to get better quality sleep enhancing the healing process.[15, 16]

Meditation: Conscious Rest

Sleep is an automatic form of unconscious rest that takes place in a state of physical and mental inactivity. Meditation – another form of rest – takes place in an active, conscious manner. Although meditation has a stigma of being a strange, mystical form of religious practice, this is far from the truth.

Meditation is a simple method of enhancing healing, relieving stress and tension, improving organ function, and expanding mental awareness and capacity. By incorporating five to 20 minutes of silent meditation in your lifestyle twice a day, you will feel the benefits immediately. After a few days, you will experience more relaxation and peace of mind. After a few weeks, you will notice changes in your body function. After a few months, you will truly know that positive changes are occurring in all areas of your life.[17]

Here is a simple meditation that is easy to incorporate into your lifestyle, providing the benefits that meditation offers. Practice this technique for five minutes twice a day, increasing a few minutes each day until you are meditating 20 minutes twice a day. The best time to meditate is immediately upon rising in the morning, preferably during sunrise and in the late afternoon just before dinner, between 4:00 and 6:00 p.m..

The Breath Meditation:

1. Sit in a comfortable position someplace quiet where you will not be disturbed.
2. Close your eyes and take 3 deep breaths allowing your body to relax. Let go of any areas that feel tight or restricted.
3. Once you feel sufficiently relaxed, put your mental attention entirely on your breath. Feel the breath going in and out of your nostrils. Feel your chest and abdomen rising and falling with the tide of the breath. Hear the sound of the breath like an ocean tide.
4. If a thought enters your mind, acknowledge it and bring your attention back to your breath.
5. Continue for five to 20 minutes. When you are finished, bring your attention back to your body. Wiggle your toes and fingers. Stretch your limbs. Slowly open your eyes and stand up.

Not only is meditation a wonderful technique for healing, stress reduction, and peace of mind, it is also a wonderful time to listen for inner guidance, intuitive solutions to challenges, and to receive creative ideas. Meditate regularly and consistently for wonderful benefits of healing and evolution.

Prayer and Thanksgiving

When I mention prayer, many people are taken aback with thoughts of religion and dogma. When I speak of prayer, I am referring to taking the time to declare to the world that which you wish to create in your life. It is a time each day to give thanks for the things we have and acknowledge the wonderment and awesomeness of our world and ourselves in a powerful form of rest; a time that allows us to separate ourselves from the hustle-bustle of everyday life. It is a time to affirm our goals and declare our vision.

Meditation is a form of silence and a moment of listening; prayer is a time to declare to the world our deepest desires and strongest intentions. It is during this time of prayer that we do the mental exercises we spoke of in chapter 8. Take time each day to affirm your vision and give thanks for the things you have and the things that are on their way. Through this moment of gratitude and intention the clear path to healing is complete.

In summary, *A Clear Path to Healing* is a series of seven responsibilities which lead the way to optimum health and wellness.

By first creating a healthy, positive mindset we set the stage for a life of optimum health. With our mind on the path to health, we focus on that which allows our mind to express itself in the physical – the nervous system.

Through spinal hygiene, freeing our spine and nervous system of tension and interference, our body and mind function optimally allowing us to live to our fullest potential. Once our nervous system is functioning at its peak, we focus on how we are nourishing our body.

By feeding our body food and drink that are water rich and free of toxicity, and filling our lungs – breathing – with oxygen-rich air, our body receives the fuel and nutrients necessary for perfect function.

By exercising our body every day, we begin to get stronger and more energized. With our new-found vibrant life, we now have energy to share with others.

Through loving relationships, our life is filled with meaning and purpose. By serving others and helping the world become a happier, healthier place, our lives are richer and we can finish each day with a well-deserved rest in an attitude of gratitude and joy.

1. Barr, M. L., M.D. Kiernan, J. A., M.D., *The Human Nervous System*, J. B. Lippincott Co., Philadelphia, 1988, pp.376-385.
2. Palmer, D.D., *The Chiropractor's Adjuster*, 1910.
3. "What is Network," http://www.networkchiropractic.org/anchomepage.htm.
4. Baylock, Russel L., *Excitotoxins: The Taste That Kills*, Health Press, 1996.
5. Martini, Betty, "World Environment Conference and the Multiple Sclerosis Foundation & FDA is Sueing For Collusion of Monsento," *Women's Cancer Research Center*, Minneapolis, 2000.
6. Raven, P., Johnson, G., *Biology*, Times Mirror/Mosby, St. Louis, 1986.
7. Wang, Sang, *Reverse Aging*, Siloam Enterprises, 1994, p. 68.
8. Wang, ibid.
9. Keith, R.E., Wade, L., "Sports Nutrition For Young Adults: Hydration," Alabama Cooperative Extension System, HE-749, New May 1997, http://www.aces.edu/department/extcomm/publications/he/he-749/he-749.html.
10. Gleick, James, *Chaos: Making a New Science*, Penguin USA, 1998.
11. Field, T., S. Schanberg, F. Scafidi, et al. 1986. Tactile/kinesthetic stimulation effects on preterm neonates. Pediatrics 77:654--658.
12. R.M. Nerem, M.J. Levesque, and J.F. Cornhill, "Social Environment As a Factor in Diet-Induced Atherosclerosis," Science 208: 1475-1476, 1980.
13. C.D.Jenkins, "Psychological and Social Precursors of Coronary Disease," *The New England Journal of Medicine* 284: 244-255, 1971.
14. "No rest for Many Weary Americans," *USA Today*, February 2, 1999.
15. "Magnetic Research and Library Information," http://www.5pillars.com/content/Mind/index.cfm?url=MagneticResearch5-24-2000.html.
16. Wang, ibid., pp. 79-89.
17. Roth, Robert, *TM Transcendental Meditation : A New Introduction to Maharishi's Easy, Effective and Scientifically Proven Technique for Promoting Better Health*, Donald L. Fine, 1994.

The Seven Healing Steps : Summary

1. **Positive Mind Cultivation** – Our thoughts create our reality. We want our minds filled with positive images of our ideal healthy self and everything we want in our life.

2. **Spinal Hygiene** – Our nervous system controls all body functions and coordinates, inspires, and heals every cell of our body. It is vital that our nervous system be free of tension and interference so that there is a clear transmission of life energy through our nerves. Chiropractic care is the most effective way to maintain a healthy spine.

3. **Clean Food and Drink** – There are seven principles for eating and drinking which provide the fuel and nutrition we need to keep our body clean of toxins.

4. **Full and Deep Breathing** – Take time each day to take 10 deep and complete breaths. The breath is the gateway to our inner healer. It provides vital oxygen, removes toxic wastes, and is an avenue to release tension and stress from our body and mind.

5. **Proper Exercise** – All life grows through movement and challenge. If we don't use it we lose. Take time each week to exercise your body.

6. **Loving Relationships** – It is through love that all things are created. If you wish to heal and experience optimum health it is vital that you love yourself and others.

7. **Adequate Rest** – In order to recover from strenuous activity and the challenges of life, we must get adequate rest. The four types of rest are Sleep, Meditation, Prayer, and Thanksgiving.

MY WISH FOR YOU

The greatest gift you can give another is to accept and receive their gift.
~ Nick Gordon

It has been a great joy and honor to share with you my truth. In expressing these words to you throughout the book I have enlightened you to a path for healing. In closing, it is important that I clarify that this is not *the* truth, nor is it *the* path to healing. For every person who walks on this earth, there lies a different truth, and for every life that passes on this planet, there lies a different path. What I have shared with you in this book comes from studying some of the truths and paths of hundreds of teachers and masters that have walked this earth, and that have been effective for millions of people around the world.

If you accept but one of the principles we explored in these pages and began to implement only one of the practices, you will experience great benefits and wonderful changes in your life. If you accept and practice all, you will create a life of optimum health and well-being, and manifest in your life all the things of which you now only dream.

I thank you for allowing me to give you my gift, for in receiving it you have given me the greatest gift of all ... that which I have always wanted ... what I *really* wanted ... to express myself to you and share with you my truth.

I thank you with all my heart.

May you be blessed with Happiness, Health, Love, Prosperity and may all your dreams, visions, goals, and intentions become real for you speedily, easily, and effortlessly.

Your friend in health,
Dr. Barry Weinberg.

DR. BARRY'S SUGGESTED READING LIST

These books have transformed my life. I recommend them to anyone who wishes to reach their optimum potential. Remember, reading provides the knowledge, but wisdom and results come from acting upon what you have learned.

All books are available online at our website: www.placeforhealing.com

Healing

Bragg, Paul and Patricia	. . . The Bragg Healthy Lifestyle
Chopra, Deepak, MD	. . . Quantum Healing Perfect Health
	The Seven Spiritual Laws of Success
Epstein, Donald, DC	. . . The 12 Stages of Healing
	Healing Myths Healing Magic
Hartmann, Thom	. . . The Last Hours of Ancient Sunlight
Kelder, Peter	. . . The Ancient Secret of the Fountain of Youth
Liedloff, Jean	. . . The Continuum Concept
Myss, Caroline	. . . Anatomy of the Spirit
	. . . Why People Don't Heal and Why They Can
Pert, Candice	. . . Molecules of Emotion
Robbins, John	. . . Diet for a New America

New Science

Capra, Frijof	. . . The Tao of Physics
Gerber, Richard, MD	. . . Vibrational Medicine
Talbot, Michael	. . . The Holographic Universe
Wilber, Ken	. . . A Brief History of Everything
Zukav, Gary	. . . The Dancing Wu Li Masters
	. . . Seat of the Soul

Immunizations, Vaccinations, and other Medical Illusions

Coulter, Harris L., PhD and Fisher, Barbara Loe	. . . A Shot in the Dark
Cournoyer, Cynthia	. . . What About Immunizations
Fisher, Barbara Loe	. . . The Consumer's Guide to Childhood
James, Walene	. . . Immunization: The Reality Behind the Illusion
Mendelsohn, Robert S.	. . . Confessions of a Medical Heretic
	. . . How to Raise a Healthy Child ... In Spite of Your Doctor
Miller, Neil Z.	. . . Immunization: Theory Vs. Reality
	. . . Immunization: The People Speak
	. . . Vaccines: Are They Really Safe and Effective
Robbins, John	. . . Reclaiming our Health

Success and Prosperity

Allen, Marc	. . . A Visionary Life
Clason, George	. . . The Richest Man in Babylon
Dyer, Wayne	. . . Manifest Your Destiny
Fisher, Marc	. . . The Instant Millionaire
Hill, Napolean	. . . Think and Grow Rich
Proctor, Bob	. . . You Were Born Rich
Ray, James A.	. . . The Science of Success
Wattles, Wallace	. . . The Science of Being Excellent
	. . . The Science of Being Healthy
	. . . The Science of Being Rich

Inspirational

	. . . The Bible
Allen, James	. . . A Heavenly Life
	. . . As A Man Thinketh
Dyer, Wayne	. . . Manifest Your Destiny
	. . . Real Magic
Fisher, Robert	. . . The Knight in Rusty Armor
Frankl, Victor	. . . Man's Search for Meaning

Inspirational (cont'd)

Gibran, Kahlil	. . . The Prophet
Hicks, Jerry and Esther	. . . A New Beginning *I, II*
Mandino, Og	. . . The Greatest Miracle in the World
	. . . The Greatest Salesman in the World
	. . . The Greatest Salesman in the World, *Part 2*
Millman, Dan	. . . Everyday Enlightenment
	. . . The Way of the Peaceful Warrior
Quinn, Daniel	. . . Ishmael
Walsch, Neale Donald	. . . Conversations with God, *Books 1, 2, 3*
	. . . Friendship with God

Motivational /Self-Empowerment

Covey, Stephen	. . . Seven Habits of Highly Effective People
Robbins, Anthony	. . . Awaken the Giant Within
	. . . Unlimited Power

———

HEALING RESOURCE GUIDE

This resource guide is a directory of organizations and web-sites for you to find support and guidance on your healing path.

A Place for Healing
   3019 NW 60th Street, Fort Lauderdale, Florida 33309
   T: (954) 970-5177
   <www.placeforhealing.com>
   drbarry@placeforhealing.com

—————

CHIROPRACTIC

Association for Network Chiropractic
   444 N. Main Street, Longmont, Colorado 80501
   T: (303) 678-8086
   <www.networkchiropractic.org>
   <www.donaldepstein.com>
   <www.innateintelligence.com>
   Research, articles, and information about Chiropractic, Network Spinal Analysis, and the 12 Stages of Healing

International Chiropractic Pediatric Association
   5295 Highway 78, Suite #D362, Stone Mountain, GA 30087-3414
   T: (770) 982-9037
   <www.4icpa.org>
   The I.C.P.A., a non-profit organization, provides information, training and research in the field of chiropractic pediatrics. The I.C.P.A. is an independent, non-political organization, and is not affiliated with any other national organization. A great resource for health research for children.

World Chiropractic Alliance
2950 N. Dobson Road, Suite 1, Chandler, AZ 85224
T: 800-347-1011
F: (602) 732-9313
<www.chiropage.com>
An incredible amount of information and resources about chiropractic
and health-care issues.

Chiro.org
<www.chiro.org/places/home.shtml>
A wonderful resource for access to health news and articles, chiropractic
research, patient information, and link categories arranged by topic.

VACCINATIONS AND
HEALTH CONSUMER AWARENESS

National Vaccine Information Center
512 W. Maple Avenue #206, Vienna, Virginia 22180
T: 1-800- 909-SHOT
<www.909shot.com>
Operated by Dissatisfied Parents Together (DPT), a national nonprofit
educational organization representing thousands of parents and health-
care professionals concerned about childhood diseases and vaccines. The
center provides support to help educate parents about vaccine safety and
their right to choose immunizations, as well as support for parents and
families who have experienced the devastation of a vaccine reaction,
injury or death. They offer books, a newsletter, information on state
vaccine laws, resource studies, lists of lawyers handling vaccine issues,
etc.

Center for Empirical Medicine
Harris L. Coulter, Ph.D., Founder
4221 45th Street N.W. , Washington, D.C. 20016, USA.
T: (202) 364 0898
F: (202) 362 3407

Center for Empirical Medicine (cont'd)
Dedicated to publicizing alternative medical thinking and to the public's right to information and choice of treatments, including (but not limited to) vaccinations.

Cancer & AIDS Cover-Up
Neil Deoul, Ph.D., Founder
<www.cancer-coverup.com>
Read this and you will never feel the same about Cancer Treatments ... Politics ... or Medical Research. Learn about the use of Cesium and Aloe to cure Cancer and AIDS ... the phenomenal results ... and their cover-up by the government and the pharmaceutical companies.

Vaccine Information & Awareness (VIA)
Karin Schumacher, Director
792 Pineview Drive, San Jose, CA 95117
T/F: (408) 554-9053
<www.access1.net/via>

Global Vaccine Awareness League
11875 Pigeon Pass Rd. #B-14-223, Moreno Valley, CA 92557
T: (909) 247-4910
<www.gval.com>

People for Reason In Science and Medicine (PRISM)
PO Box 2102, Anaheim, CA 92814
T: (805) 255-9522
A nonprofit health and environmental organization.

Vaccination Alternatives
P.O. Box 346, New York, NY 10023
T: (212) 890-5117
Director: Sharon Kimmelman

ALKALINE WATER

Alkazone
> c/o Better Health Labs, Inc.
> 221 – 62nd St., W. New York, NJ 07093
> T: 1-800-810-1888
> <www.alkazone.com>

MAGNETIC AND FAR-INFRARED PRODUCTS

Wellness & Success
> Anja Weinberg, Independent Nikken Distributor
> <anja.5pillars.com>
> E-mail: anja@5pillars.com

OTHER HEALING RESOURCES

Transcendental Meditation
> <www.tm.org>
> A simple, natural, effortless technique for reducing stress and developing an individual's full mental and physical potential. It is easily-learned and practiced for 15-20 minutes twice a day, sitting comfortably with the eyes closed.

Deepak Chopra's Website
> <www.chopra.com>
> A wonderful website with information and products pertaining to healing and specifically, *Ayurveda*, an ancient Indian health-care system.

Holistic Online
> <www.holistic-online.com>
> A comprehensive, interactive and objective web site about your health choices featuring alternative medicine and modern western medicine.

Earthmed.com
> <www.earthmed.com>
> An online directory of holistic practitioners, organizations and products.

OneBody.com
  <www.onebody.com>
  An online community dedicated to connecting people with healthy
  alternatives and healing professionals.

POLITICAL, SPIRITUAL
AND AWARENESS RESOURCES

Global Renaissance Alliance
  P.O. Box 15712, Washington D.C. 20003
  T: (202) 544-1219
  F: (202) 347-0544
  <www.renaissancealliance.org>
  The Global Renaissance Alliance seeks to create a dynamic context for
  the marriage of spiritual and political pursuits. They provide the
  encouragement and tools for American citizens to actively participate in
  the Democratic process from a space, which honors body, mind and
  spirit.

The Natural Law Party
  1946 Mansion Drive, P.O. Box 1900, Fairfield, IA 52556
  T: (515) 472-2040
  <www.natural-law.org>
  <www.hagelin.org>
  The Natural Law Party holds that natural law is the solution to problems.
  Government can solve problems at their basis through scientifically
  proven programs to bring every citizen, and the entire nation, into accord
  with natural law. By accessing the full range of nature's intelligence and
  harnessing its power, individuals and nations can govern themselves with
  the same perfection in administration displayed throughout nature.

Re-Creation
  1257 Siskiyou Blvd., #1150, Ashland, OR 97520
  T: (541) 482-8806
  <www.conversationswithgod.org>
  A foundation focused on personal growth and spiritual understanding
  created by Neale Donald Walsch, author of the *Conversation with God*
  book series.

GLOSSARY

Acceptance	(*Latin, to take*) 1. to receive willingly whatever is present in the moment regardless if it is uncomfortable, inconvenient, or undesired. 2. one of the seven "Processes of the Heart" 3. one of the seven "Powers of the Mind."
Acid Food	(*Latin, sour*) any food that produces an acidic condition in the body. All disease processes occur in an acidic environment. Acidic foods are all meats, grains, nuts, seeds, and "junk" foods. Exceptions are salmon, millet, and almonds. A healthy diet should consist of less than 25% acid foods.
Acknowledgment	(*Latin, to know*) 1. to declare that something is so; to recognize and declare your own or another's talent, ability, or authority. 2. one of the seven "Processes of the Heart."
Adaptability	(*French, to fit*) 1. the ability to effectively and efficiently adjust oneself internally to changes in the outside world in such a way as to prevent adverse effects to your body or mind. 1. one of the seven "Attributes of Health."
Addiction	(*Latin, to give assent*) an irresistible craving for a substance, activity, emotion, or thought that is detrimental to the body and mind, yet is believe to bring increased joy, peace, or freedom.
Affirmation	(*Latin, to make firm*) 1. a declaration said out loud or quietly to oneself that something is so. 2. one of the seven "Processes of the Heart" 3. one of the seven "Powers of the Mind."

Alkaline Food

(*Arabic, the qili – ash of a saltwort plant*) any food that produces an alkaline condition in the body. A healthy body exists in an environment. Alkaline foods are all fruits and vegetables, with the exception of pomegranites. A healthy diet should consist of more than 75% alkaline foods.

Allopathic Model

(*Greek, other suffering*) the current model of health-care utilized and promoted by the medical profession which encourages the treatment of disease using chemicals, radiation, or surgery to produce effects that are opposite to those produced by the disease. i.e. taking pain killers to alleviate headaches or blood pressure medication to lower elevated blood pressure.

Allowance

(*Latin, to a place*) 1. to give oneself permission to experience whatever sensation, event, thought, or emotion that arises in order to achieve a desired result. 2. one of the seven "Powers of the Mind."

Anger

(*Old Norse, distress*) 1. a feeling of displeasure and hostility resulting from an event in which one felt dishonored, disrespected, opposed, or harmed in some way. 2. one of the seven "Emotions of Healing."

Antibiotic

(*Greek, against life*) a substance that destroys or stops the growth of living cells, whether bacterial, botanical, animal or human.

Anxiety

(*Latin, to choke*) 1. an uneasiness about what may occur in the future. 2. one of the seven "Emotions of Healing."

Apathy

(*French, without emotion*) 1. not caring about what has occurred in the past, what is occurring in the present, or what may occur in the future. 2. one of the seven "Causes of the Health-Care Crisis" 3. one of the seven "Emotions of Healing."

Atom

(*Greek, uncut*) an infinitesimally small collection of energy particles organized in the form of a solar system that constitute the foundation upon which the physical world is constructed.

Atonement	(*Middle English, at one*) 1. OLD DEFINITION – to make amends for a wrongdoing. 2. NEW DEFINITION (At-One-Ment) – to become aware of, experience, and express your unity with all things in the universe. 3. one of the seven "Processes of the Heart."
Awareness	(*Old English, cautious*) 1. to know, realize, or be conscious of. 2. one of the seven "Processes of the Heart."
Awe	(*Old Norse, awe*) 1. a mixed feeling of reverence, love, and wonder. 2. one of the seven "Processes of the Heart."
Belief	(*Old English, belief*) 1. a certainty that something is true. 2. one of the seven "Powers of the Mind."
Cell	(*Latin, small room*) 1. a microscopic mass of water, proteins, carbohydrates and fats surrounded by a membrane capable of performing all of life's functions alone or with other cells.; 2. the fundamental structure upon which all living things are constructed.
Cerebrospinal Fluid	(*Latin, brain + thorn + to flow*) a nutrient rich fluid that flows through the brain and spinal cord providing them with circulation, protection, and nutrition.
Chiropractic	(*Greek, done by hand*) a philosophy, science, and art that detects, analyzes, and corrects vertebral subluxations. (see Vertebral Subluxation).
Contentment	(*Latin, to hold together*) 1. the experience of feeling satisfied. 2. one of the seven "Attributes of Health."
Craving	(*Old English, crave*) an intense longing or hunger, usually for something the body or mind needs. (see Addiction)
Creativity	(*Latin, create*) 1. the ability to bring into existence something (an idea, object, image, sound, etc.) that did not exist before. 2. one of the seven "Powers of the Mind."

Curing	(*Latin, care*) the use of a substance, procedure, or energy to return the body or mind to a state of normal or average. (see Healing)
Decision	(*Latin, to cut off*) 1. to make up one's mind towards one possibility distinct from all others. 2. one of the seven "Powers of the Mind."
Desire	(*French, from a star*) 1. "a possibility seeking expression or a function seeking performance." – Wallace Wattles, *The Science of Getting Rich* 2. one of the seven "Powers of the Mind."
Discrimination	(*Latin, to separate apart*) 1. to distinguish the differing qualities or properties of two objects, experiences, or ideas. 2. one of the seven "Powers of the Mind."
Disease	(*Latin, not lying nearby*) 1. an experience of degeneration, dysfunction, or discomfort in the body or mind; 2. an absence of ease. (see Ease)
DNA	(*Deoxyribonucleic Acid*) 1. an essential component of all living things that provides the genetic information for development and function of the body and mind; 2. the molecule that transmits genetic information from one generation to the next within one species of bacteria, plant or animal.
Doubt	(*Latin, to doubt*) 1. a condition of uncertainty or disbelief. 2. one of the seven "Emotions of Healing."
Dura Mater	(*Latin, tough mother*) 1. a durable membrane that surrounds the brain and spinal cord housing the cerebrospinal fluid and providing further protection to the nervous system; 2. the outer layer of the meninges. (see Cerebrospinal fluid, meninges)
Ease	(*Latin, lying nearby*) 1. a state of peace, well-being, and contentment; 2. to be free of tension or pressure.
Elan Vital	(*French, rushing life*) life force; nerve energy; chi; prana.

Energy   (*Greek, in work*) force of expression; inherent power; capacity for action.

Environment   (*Greek, in a circuit*) all the conditions, circumstances, and factors (biological, ecological, cultural, etc.) surrounding and effecting the development of a living thing.

Evolution   (*Latin, to roll out*) 1. the ability to adapt to a long-term or permanent change in the environment. 2. an unfolding process of development; the process of becoming more – more intelligent, more efficient, more capable, etc. 3. one of the seven "Attributes of Health."

Exercise   (*Latin, to put to work*) to place stress on the body or mind with the purpose of becoming stronger, more flexible, and more capable.

Expression   (*Latin, to press out*) 1. the ability to manifest physically a mental intention. 2. the outward announcement of an idea, feeling, or attribute through art (thought), sound (word), or behavior (deed). 3. one of the seven "Attributes of Health."

Faith   (*Latin, to trust*) 1. the knowing that something is so without any evidence. 2. one of the seven "Powers of the Mind."

Far-Infrared   (*Latin, far below red*) 1. invisible rays of the light spectrum that is given off by the human body as heat; 2. the nurturing, life sustaining rays of the sun, as opposed to ultraviolet.

Fear   (*Old English, danger*) 1. the absence of love; 2. the experience of expecting danger or hardship in the near future. 3. one of the seven "Emotions of Healing.

Fight or Flight   (*Old English*) an automatic defense mechanism of living things preparing it for confrontation or retreat from a real or imagined danger.

Germ Theory	(*Latin, sprout*) a belief originated, and eventually dismissed, by Louis Pasteur that all diseases are caused by destructive external agents called germs, i.e. bacteria and viruses.
Gratitude	(*Latin, thankful*) 1. an experience of feeling thankful appreciation for things received. 2. one of the seven "Powers of the Mind."
Harmonious Interaction	(*Greek, fitting + doing together*) 1. the ability to have peaceful relationships with others 2. a peaceful, interdependent, mutually benefiting relationship between two beings. 3. one of the seven "Attributes of Health."
Healing	(*Old English, whole*) 1. the process by which a "whole" that has lost its integrity becoming separate, disconnected, damaged, harmed or shamed, regains its wholeness; 2. the process by which we regain health.
Health	(*Old English, whole*) 1. the experience of complete physical, mental, emotional, social, and spiritual well-being, ease, and freedom, and not merely the absence of disease, pain or symptoms. 2. the ability to effectively and efficiently perceive change, adapt to change, recover from change, grow from the experience, express physically a mental intention, harmoniously interact with others, and experience contentment. 3. a joyful, peaceful, love-filled and free experience of life; and a full expression of who you are and the unique gifts you have to offer the world.
Helplessness	(*Old English, without help*) 1. the feeling that one is powerless to change one's current circumstance, situation, or experience. 2. one of the seven "Illusions of Disease."
Illusion	(*Latin, to mock*) an idea, perception, or image that appears real, but isn't.
Imagination	(*Latin, to image*) 1. the mental ability to form mental images, create new ideas, and invent possible futures. 2. one of the seven "Powers of the Mind."

Immune System   (*Latin, without duties*) a complex system within all living things that protects the body from outside agents which would have otherwise been detrimental. (note: Disease is a result of the body's inability to respond to these outside agents effectively, rather than the agents themselves.)

Immunization   (*Latin, without duties*) the process by which one becomes immune to a substance, organism, or circumstance. (see Vaccination)

Inclusive Evolution   (*Latin, to close in + to roll out*) 1. the natural law that states that the whole is always greater than its parts; and that all things that are individual are always a part of something greater, including ourselves. 2. one of the seven "Universal Principles of Healing."

Innate Intelligence   (*Latin, in born + choose between*) the inborn quality within all living things that controls and coordinates all body function, inspires, and heals.

Integrity   (*Latin, whole*) completeness; wholeness.

Intelligence   (*Latin, choose between*) 1. the ability to learn or understand. 2. the ability to cope with a new situation. 3. the ability to evolve, change and transform itself into higher levels of creativity, abstraction, and unpredictability. 4. degree of awareness.

Intention   (*Latin, to stretch at*) 1. a determination to be, think or act in a predetermined, specified way. 2. to have one's purpose or attention firmly fixed on a desired outcome. 3. the choosing of a desired result with the confidence that it will be. 4. one of the seven "Powers of the Mind."

Judgment   (*Latin, saying law*) 1. an opinion or belief about something. 2. one of the seven "Powers of the Mind."

Love   (*Old English*) an expression of unity in which one experiences the wonder, beauty, and uniqueness of another or oneself creating feelings of joy, compassion, peace, and freedom.

Meditation   (*Latin, to plan or intend*) a process of conscious rest in which one focuses the mind on one point (a sound, image, etc.) with the purpose of relaxing the body and quieting the mind in order to improve health, receive creative ideas and inner guidance, and achieve higher states of awareness and consciousness.

Meninges   (*Greek, membrane*) a three layer membrane that surrounds and protects the brain and spinal cord encasing the cerebrospinal fluid.

Nervous System   (*Latin*) 1. an interconnected network of energy and information transmitting fibers consisting of the brain, spinal cord and nerves that controls and coordinates all body and mind function. 2. an energy and information processing system that allows an organism to perceive and respond to its environment.

Nesting   (*Coined by Ken Wilber*) the concept by which smaller entities unite to create something greater that not only contains the properties of its constituents but acquires newer, more evolved qualities. i.e. atoms which form molecules which form cells which form a living thing.

Network Spinal Analysis   (*Coined by Dr. Donald Epstein*) a profound sequence of spinal evaluations and adjusting techniques which increases flexibility, expands inner awareness, and improves quality of life by helping the body to develop innate strategies to release stored tension and more effectively respond appropriately to stress.

Neurological Tone   (*Latin, nerve science + to stretch*) the degree of physical tension in the nerve tissue that affects the way it transmits and interprets energy and information.

Objective Dogma   (*Latin, to throw to + Greek, think*) 1. the belief that something is true only if it can be proved by the scientific method, dismissing all inner experience and unexplained phenomenon. 2. one of the seven "Causes of the Health-Care Crisis."

Paradigm   (*Greek, beside example*) one current world-view, perception, or model of reality.

Perception	(*Latin, take through*) 1. the ability to become aware of something through the senses or other means. 2. one of the seven "Attributes of Health."
Permanence	(*Latin, remain through*) 1. the state or belief that something will remain indefinitely. 2. one of the seven "Illusions of Disease."
Possession	(*Latin, have*) 1. to have or believe one has something that one owns or belongs to 2. one of the seven "Illusions of Disease."
Quantum Physics	(*Latin, how much + nature*) the scientific study of the fundamental structure of the universe and the relationship between energy and matter.
Recovery	(*Latin, to get back or regain*) 1. to return to a state of ease after adapting, responding, or being affected by a change in the environment. 2. one of the seven "Attributes of Health."
Responsibility	(*Latin, to pledge back*) the ability to consciously choose thoughts and behaviors that are in the best interest of ourselves and others, and to act upon those choices. (see Response ability)
Response Ability	(*Latin, to pledge back*) the ability to respond appropriately to changes in our internal and external environment, whether consciously or sub-consciously. (see Responsibility)
Sadness	(*Old English, sated*) 1. an unhappy feeling resulting from a real or imagined loss or lack of something 2. one of the seven "Emotions of Healing."
Segregation	(*Latin, a flock apart*) to set apart or separate an individual or group, cellularly, socially, etc. 2. one of the seven "Causes of the Health-Care Crisis."
Separation	(*Latin, to arrange apart*) 1. to break apart a whole into distinct individual parts. 2. one of the seven "Causes of the Health-Care Crisis." 3. one of the seven "Illusions of Disease."

Stress — (*Latin, strict*) a change in the outside environment that causes a change in one's internal environment, whether this change be of a physical, emotional, or chemical nature.

Subjective Creation — (*Latin, to throw under create*) 1. the principle that our experience of reality and our world, and perhaps reality itself, is a manifestation of our thoughts, perceptions, beliefs, and interpretations. 2. one of the seven "Universal Principles of Healing."

Subluxation — see Vertebral Subluxation.

Suffering — (*Latin, to bear under*) the experience of pain or loss, accompanied by sadness, helplessness, and confusion.

Symbiosis — (*Latin, to live together*) the living together of two different kinds of organisms providing mutual advantage to both.

Symptom — (*Greek, to fall together*) 1. any accompanying circumstance or condition that indicates the existence of something. 2. a mechanism of the body and mind to alert the individual of a change or a need for change, or to create a needed change.

T-Cell — an integral part of the immune system which provides immunity to the cells. This is the primary cell attacked by the AIDS virus. The "T" stands for thymus, an organ beneath the breast bone which is integral in the development of the immune system.

Tone — (*Greek, to stretch*) 1. the perceived quality, expression, character, or attitude of a given situation, environment, individual, color, sound, etc. 2. the degree of tension in something.

Unified Abundance — (*Latin, made one + to rise away in waves*) 1. the principle that although the universe appears to be made up of an infinitude of separate parts, they are in fact all aspects of one unified whole. 2. one of the seven "Universal Principles of Healing."

Unified Field	(*Latin, made one* + *Old English, field*) a theoretical field in physics from which all energy arises, including electromagnetism, gravity, and the forces that hold together atomic structures.
Universe	(*Latin, one turn*) the totality of all things that exist.
Universal Intelligence	(*Latin, one turn* + *to stretch at*) 1. that which is within all things that maintains them in existence, gives them their properties, and governs their behavior. 2. one of the seven "Universal Principles of Healing."
Unwavering Traditionalism	(*Latin, not waving* + *deliver*) 1. the concept that people tend to hold on to traditional ideas resisting change and new paradigms of belief out of a herd mentality and a fear of the unknown. 2. one of the seven "Causes of the Health-Care Crisis"
Vaccination	(*Latin, cow*) a form of artificial immunization in which a mild form of a disease (i.e. polio) is administered to a person orally or by injection with the intention that the body will produce antibodies or immune factors to protect itself from the vaccine, developing immunity to and providing protection from future exposure to the disease.
Vertebrae	(*Latin, to turn*) one of the 24 movable bones which make up the spinal column protecting the spinal cord from outside forces.
Vertebral Subluxation	(*Latin, to turn* + *condition of less light*) a condition in the spine in which there is either a build-up of tension in the spinal tissues or a malpositioned vertebrae, or both, interfering with the transmission of mental impulse through the nerves causing dysfunction, dis-ease, and eventually death.
Vibration	(*Latin, to shake*) 1. a rapid, periodic back and forth movement 2. one of the seven "Universal Principles of Healing."

Visualization

(*Latin, to cause to see*) 1. to form a mental image of something that is not present to the sight.
2. one of the seven "Powers of the Mind."

Vitalism

(*Latin, life doctrine*) 1. a doctrine that the functions of a living thing are due to a living force or energy distinct from physiological and biochemical forces. 2. a doctrine that the processes of life are self-determining and are not dictated by the laws of physics and chemistry alone, but by an intelligent force. 3. the doctrine upon which chiropractic and *A Clear Path to Healing* are based.

ABOUT THE AUTHOR

Dr. Barry S. Weinberg is the author of *A Clear Path to Healing* and chief doctor and founder of A Place for Healing in Fort Lauderdale, Florida. Dr. Barry (as his clients affectionaly call him) is a dedicated healing facilitator, teacher, writer, musician, and public speaker. He has been in private practice as a Chiropractor since 1994. He has a Bachelors degree in Nutrition, as well as a Doctorate in Chiropractic. Through his extensive studies, Dr. Barry has acquired a vast knowledge of health, psychology, physics, spirituality, and success principles.

In his efforts to educate the community, Dr. Barry gives seminars and workshops across South Florida. He has spoken in such venues as Florida Atlantic University, Unity Churches, Border's and Barnes and Noble bookstores, Whole Life Market, and many other local organizations and businesses. He has been the writer and publisher of a quarterly newsletter called *A Place for Healing News*, which has satisfied an audience of over 500 for the last 6 years. His articles have appeared in such periodicals as *The Yoga Journal, Inner Self, Ideas*, and *One Heart* magazines. Dr. Barry has recently been invited to be a board member of the Southern Chiropractic Association in which he will reside as the new editor of the SCA newsletter.

Dr. Barry is currently the Fort Lauderdale representative for an international health awareness day for children called Kid's Day America/International proclaimed an "official day" by both Mayor Jim Naugle and Governor Jeb Bush. Through this event, he has exposed hundreds of children to the importance of good health, a clean environment, and being drug free. In 2000, he raised over $2500 for Kids InDistress (a South Florida charity) through this event. He has also been the exam doctor for The Special Olympics and Project Insight for the last few years.

Dr. Barry maintains a vision for a healthy, vibrant world based on the principles of Healing, Love, Truth, and Freedom. He has dedicated his life to bringing greater awareness and healing to the public through education and chiropractic care. By acting locally and thinking globally, Dr. Barry will continue to make his vision a reality by educating the community and ...

Creating a Healthier World ... One Life at a Time.

COMING SOON

TO FACE A DRAGON

Take an adventure of self-discovery in this fairytale metaphor of the healing process we all go through. Join young Theodore as he confronts the Dragon which destroyed his village and threatened his life and discovers his own powers of healing and creation. Walk with Theodore as he meets many unique characters along the way, each representing another part of each us, including fear, doubt, courage, and our own inner voice.

A CLEAR PATH TO HEALING AUDIOCASSETTES

Enjoy listening to this enlightening book in the convenience of your home or car.

WORKSHOPS AND SEMINARS

Dr. Barry Weinberg is available for seminars and workshops, or as a keynote speaker. In addition, he encourages those who have studied his book to form study groups based on *A Clear Path to Healing*. Please visit our website at www.placeforhealing.com.

INDEX

INDEX

C

cancer, 3, 21, 35, 38, 44, 50, 82, 89, 90, 94, 111, 112, 130, 134, 139, 146, 148, 174
career, 77, 96, 104, 137
Carlin, George, 120
carnivores vs. herbivores, 152-153
cause and effect, 56, 57, 72, 75
cause of disease, 25, 26, 90
cells, 6, 26, 38, 45, 46, 48, 50, 59-64, 66, 69-71, 80, 86, 96, 145, 149, 151, 152
cerebral palsy, 44
cerebrospinal fluid, 145
certainty, 30, 118, 119, 125, 126, 140
challenge, 19, 80, 94, 121, 136, 139, 142, 149, 156, 157, 159, 163, 166
change, 10, 13, 15, 19-25, 30, 45-46, 57-58, 61, 62, 71-75, 77-84, 87-88, 89-99, 108, 111, 112, 117, 121, 126-130, 132, 134-135, 139, 144-147, 149, 150, 154, 158, 160, 163, 167
chemotherapy, 35-36
children, 27-29, 137, 152, 160, 189
Chiropractic, 129-130, 139, 146-148, 166, 172, 173, 179, 189
choice, 11, 13, 20, 29, 35, 62, 82, 96-98, 99, 104, 140
cholesterol, 5, 35, 158-159
Chopra, Deepak, MD, xiii, 45, 67, 168, 175
chronic fatigue syndrome, 147
Church, the, 24-25, 26
civilization, 80
clarity, 10, 11
codependent relationship, 47
cold, 37, 50, 162
Columbus, Christopher, 25
commitment, 103
communication, 12, 144, 145
community, 12, 19, 20, 25, 27, 34, 39, 64, 67, 77, 113
computers, 25, 60, 157
confidence, 11, 46, 87, 121
confusion, 10, 126
consciousness, 14, 64, 69, 120, 135
contentment, 77, 86-88, 135, 145, 146, 179
contradiction, 3, 22, 32, 35

contribution, 11, 104
Copernicus, 24-25
Coulter, Harris L., MD, 27, 170, 173
Cournoyer, Cynthia, 27, 170
Crack in the Cosmic Egg, the, 33
cravings, 148, 150
creation, 12, 14, 69, 72, 74, 102-103, 105, 108, 115, 139, 186
creativity, 11, 12, 64, 65, 67, 104, 115, 127, 179
creator, 29, 139
crime, 14, 15, 31, 39, 71, 86, 159
criminal rehabilitation, 39
crisis, 19-42, 46, 47, 51, 55, 73, 79, 81, 83, 84, 127
Crohn's disease, 92, 150
culture, 19, 52, 80, 90
curing, 5-6, 7, 15, 180
cyclophosphamide, 36

D

Darwin, Charles, 63
death, 3, 6, 21, 27, 28, 30, 31, 33-35, 45, 87, 90, 118, 133, 159
decision, 21, 29, 42, 91, 94, 96,105-106, 109, 115, 127, 130, 140, 180
degenerative, 3, 21, 146, 153, 154, 157
dehydration, 154
denial, 131, 132, 136, 142
depression, 13, 32, 134, 139, 146
Descartes, René, 5
desire, 2, 9, 12-15, 55-58, 61, 64, 65, 69, 74, 76, 84, 86, 87, 103, 104, 107, 110, 113, 116, 119, 133, 134, 145, 164, 180
detoxification, 162
diabetes, 3, 21, 44, 84, 89, 146
diagnosis, 5, 44
diarrhea, 37, 48, 57
Dickey, Nancy, MD, 3
diet, 21, 23, 79, 134, 135, 146, 149, 151, 153, 154
differentiation, 69
digestion, 63, 91, 149-150, 161
diptheria, 28
discovery, 14, 25, 33, 98
discrimination, 106-107, 115, 180
dis-ease, 21, 42, 52, 66, 73, 92, 96, 111, 117, 120-122, 125, 130, 156, 160

Give the Gift of
A Clear Path to Healing

to your loved ones, friends, clients and colleagues!

Check your leading bookstore or order here.

YES, I would like to order _____ copies of

A Clear Path to Healing

Quantity	Price	Total Cost
1-9	$14.95	
10 - 25	$14.50	
25 - 30	$13.95	
50 +	$10.00	
Subtotal		
6.5% Tax (Florida only)		
Shipping: $3.75 first book, $.75 ea. addn'l		
Total		

Name _____

Organization _____

Street Address _____

City _____ State _____ Zip Code _____

Telephone _____ Fax _____

E-mail _____

Method of Payment: ❑ VISA   ❑ MASTERCARD   ❑ DISCOVER
❑ CHECK - Made payable to: A Place for Healing
Mail to: 3019 N W 60th Street
Fort Lauderdale, Florida, 33309

Credit card number _____

Expiry date: _____

Cardholder signature:_____

**For faster service, call 1-800-715-4788, fax (954) 970-4587 or
e-mail: drbarry@placeforhealing.com. Allow 15 days for delivery.**